# Conflicts in Care
## Medicine and Nursing

*Lesley Mackay*

Senior Research Fellow
Department of Applied Social Science
Lancaster University
UK

**CHAPMAN & HALL**

London · Glasgow · New York · Tokyo · Melbourne · Madras

**Published by Chapman & Hall, 2–6 Boundary Row, London SE1 8HN**

Chapman & Hall, 2–6 Boundary Row, London SE1 8HN, UK

Blackie Academic & Professional, Wester Cleddens Road, Bishopbriggs, Glasgow G64 2NZ, UK

Chapman & Hall, 29 West 35th Street, New York NY10001, USA

Chapman & Hall Japan, Thomson Publishing Japan, Hirakawacho Nemoto Building, 6F, 1–7–11 Hirakawa-cho, Chiyoda-ku, Tokyo 102, Japan

Chapman & Hall Australia, Thomas Nelson Australia, 102 Dodds Street, South Melbourne, Victoria 3205, Australia

Chapman & Hall India, R. Seshadri, 32 Second Main Road, CIT East, Madras 600 035, India

Distributed in the USA and Canada by Singular Publishing Group Inc., 4284 41st Street, San Diego, California 92105

First edition 1993

© 1993 Lesley Mackay

Typeset in Palatino 10/12 pt by Columns Design & Production Services Ltd, Reading
Printed in Great Britain by Clays Ltd, Bungay, Suffolk

ISBN 0 412 47860 9      1 56593 120 3 (USA)

A catalogue record for this book is available from the British Library

Library of Congress Cataloging-in-Publication data available

# Contents

# Acknowledgements

Many people have contributed to the making of this book. Without the help of the many nurses and doctors who were interviewed, the book could not have been written; to them I give my warmest thanks.

Because the locations in which the research was undertaken must remain anonymous, those many helpful people who ensured that the research went ahead must also remain anonymous, but their contribution must be acknowledged.

As directors of the research team, thanks must go to Professor Keith Soothill and Dr Sylvia Walby. Especial thanks to Keith Soothill for keeping the show on the road. The research was funded by the Economic and Social Research Council (Research Award Number R000 23 1394) and whose support is gratefully acknowledged.

The tedious task of transcribing interviews fell to Gail Nutter, Mary-Ann McKerchar, Janet Chapman, Ann Anderton, and Ros Platt. Thanks must also go to Chris Quinn who always dealt calmly with my panics over a word-processor which had a will of its own.

I would also like to thank Wilhelmina Mills for her kind permission to let me quote from her unpublished Masters thesis: a work which deserves attention.

My particular thanks must be reserved for June Greenwell who as part of our research team and a nursing professional provided many valuable insights, great encouragement and an unfailing sense of humour while the work progressed. Her comments on the manuscript were particularly helpful.

Lesley Mackay
1993

# 1

# Playing the game

We are all familiar with the game called 'Doctors and Nurses'. From our earliest days we used to play it: as doctor or nurse. As 'patients' being bandaged and administered to, we learned what was required of us. We were told 'doctor knows best' and that 'the nurse will look after you'. We knew not to believe them when they said it wouldn't hurt, but we joined in the game. It prepared us for real life where we learned other things to expect: the waiting in corridors and ante-rooms, the quiescence of not speaking until we are spoken to, the need to sit still, the gratefulness for the attentions we receive. The special feel of the hospital, of hushed activity and serious matters is an integral part of our understanding of how our health needs are attended to. To some extent, then, most of us have been doctors and nurses and all of us will be patients.

### RELIANCE AND TRUST

We rely heavily on hospitals and medical science. Our demands for the services which hospitals offer seems to be insatiable. Yet we have fears and apprehensions about the treatment. We need the game to be played. None of us is that certain about medical science and the techniques and procedures that need to be performed in order to restore us to health. We are unsure about things being done to us that might hurt and cause us discomfort and pain.

We have to trust the people who work in hospitals. We have to feel they are doing the best they can for us. If we are distrustful and suspicious, then our emotional commitment to our treatment is impaired and our recovery delayed or made impossible. We need to believe, and nurses and doctors make it their business to maintain our belief in hospitals, in medical science, and in their capacity to help us. We also need to feel that they know what one another is doing and that they work as a team for the benefit of their patients.

What lies behind the united and agreeable front which doctors and nurses present to us? Do they have fights and if so, what do they fight about? What weapons do they use? Why don't we hear about these fights? Who is the winner and who is the loser? How does this affect the care that they give? Perhaps nurses and doctors should stand back from their own working perspective and consider a broader picture of what they do.

## IDENTIFYING CONFLICT

From previous research I had carried out with Keith Soothill, it had been revealed that there were conflicts between nurses and doctors (Mackay, 1989). This research had also suggested what these conflicts may have been about and why they occurred. But further investigation was needed to explore the working relationships between doctors and nurses. Funding was gratefully received from the Economic and Social Research Council (Award No. R000 23 1394) and the research was embarked on in early 1989 (Appendix A).

### Focusing the research

The hospital is the sieve through which every nurse and doctor proceeds. It is in the hospital environment that each learns their own place. It is within the hospital that attitudes towards members of the other group are formed and remain influential (Bowling, 1981, p.31). Hospital health care dominates the National Health Service and the way in which our health care needs are defined and attended to. Closer examination of the hospital's inside may help explain what happens on its outside.

It was obvious that relationships would be different in each specialty and that they would be experienced differently by the varying grades of nurses and doctors. It was decided to focus on five specialties: general medicine, general surgery, intensive therapy, mental illness and medicine for the elderly.

Access to hospitals in five locations was obtained. Some of these, however, had insufficient beds, and therefore also insufficient nurses and doctors, in some of the our chosen specialties. In these hospitals, two other specialties were chosen: otolaryngology and paediatrics. From the end of 1989 right through 1990, a total of 262 doctors and nurses were interviewed by June Greenwell and myself (Appendix B).

June and I got to know the hospitals very well. Two were teaching hospitals: one in London and the other in Scotland. Three were district general hospitals: one in Scotland, one in the north and one in the south of England. They were very different from one another yet, curiously, the same. NHS hospitals have a common yet distinctive feel to them: the echoes of their corridors; the kiosks and the canteens; the colours and the smells; the ambulancemen hanging around the entrance; the reception desk and the usual inexplicable signpostings to the wards. There is nowhere else quite like a hospital; as an organization it is unique and it is a special place in which to work.

## THE WORK FORCE

Thousands of people work in each hospital: cleaners, nurses, physiotherapists, porters, radiologists, doctors, technicians, maintenance men and ladies pushing trolleys. Choosing to interview only nurses and doctors is not to ignore the contributions and perspectives of all the others who take part in the provision of health care in hospitals. However, in what was an exploratory investigation it was necessary to limit the focus of attention. The decision was taken to concentrate on trained nurses and doctors rather than students and un-qualified nursing staff. All grades of doctors were inter-viewed, from recently qualified house officers to consultants and two levels of nurses: Staff Nurses and Sister/Charge Nurses.

### Interview techniques

Because many of the nurses and doctors were interviewed at work, this meant that it was not always possible to complete the planned hour-long interview. Interruptions and emergency calls meant that some interviews were considerably shorter than others. In other cases, particularly when interviews were conducted after working hours, on the night shift, or in the respondent's home, the interview might be substantially longer. This means that the number of responses for each topic area varies.

Also, because this was exploratory research, semi-structured interviews were used. Questionnaires were felt to be inappropriate on a subject which might be both emotive and highly personal. While there were a number of topic areas we sought to cover in each interview, items of particular interest or relevance to the respondent would be followed up in greater detail. And as the interview programme progressed, additional topics of interest emerged which became part of the 'core' questions asked. Again, this means that there is a variation in the level of response to each question.

The identities of the kind and accommodating people who agreed to share their experiences regarding inter-profession relations must be protected. Both they and the locations in which the interviews took place will remain anonymous. However, the grade of the person will be given and other information such as specialty, location or gender only noted where relevant to the argument being presented. Because it is simpler, nurses will be referred to as female and doctors as male, even although nearly half of medical students are female. A natural association is made by nurses and doctors along these lines. Only occasionally was this automatic association of the gender of colleagues in the other occupation qualified.

## Using the data

Although I shall use some accumulated data from the interviews these should not be accorded disproportionate interest. The nurses and doctors who have to work together are constantly moving. Colleagues change from month to month; nurses and junior doctors move from specialty to specialty. Their comments, therefore, reflect their own individual working experiences. Aggregated data can, therefore, have only limited applicability. The specific concerns and comments of each individual are part of his or her own particular perspective.

Combining the comments of many individuals on any one topic may be, therefore, both dubious and unreliable. Nevertheless some tabular information will be provided in the appendices for those who like such data and to try to avoid the danger of sailing too close to mere literature about which Lepenies (1988) warns sociologists.

At the same time, it has to be remembered that in acting as individuals, we also act as members of a group. The identities gained from membership of a professional group can be particularly influential in affecting what we respond to and how we respond to others. Discussion of 'the group' is therefore of interest because the group may inform our actions. Similarly, over-emphasis on the group may obscure the day-to-day working together of nurses and doctors. All of us fit into some group, but the degree of that 'fit' varies. Neither doctors nor nurses are homogenous groups of people. The problems of generalizing were pointed out by Wilson (1954, p.10): 'every operating room is: (a) like **all** other operating rooms (b) like **some** other operating rooms (c) like **no** other operating rooms'. There are many other considerations which make generalizations difficult. At a minimum, consideration has to be given to both professional and individual influences on behaviour and to try to identify tensions between the two.

Generalizations can be helpful in describing trends, but they do not describe the situations facing individuals and for this reason may fail to 'resonate' with practitioners' own experiences. The particular and special experiences of the nurses and doctors who were interviewed have to be obscured both to protect their anonymity and to avoid the potentially idiosyncratic nature of their view of the world. Each individual faces a situation which to a greater or lesser degree is different from that facing any other individual. For every grade of staff, within each ward or unit, within each speciality, within each hospital, within each region and each country there there will be differences in the situation they face. To follow the so-called 'scientific method' which aggregates individuals' comments is a way in which individualities can be ignored (Lepenies, 1988, p.150). Nevertheless, in writing this book it has been necessary to stand back from the hard-working and helpful individuals who were interviewed and take a cooler look at the issues underlying their comments and observations.

### 'Normal' and 'abnormal' responses

In considering the accounts of nurses and doctors, it must be emphasized that what is remembered in people's accounts of their world is the abnormal: the normal goes unnoticed just because it is normal. If, in this book, there is too great a reliance on the difficulties, that is because they help identify the issues which shape the way members of different occupational groups relate to one another at work. In artificially abstracting two or three 'interesting' comments on a particular topic from an individual's account, the integrity of what they are saying may be lost. Thus, a couple of acerbic comments from an otherwise contented individual can easily give the wrong impression. At the same time, it is often easier to moan about than to praise colleagues and the opportunity to 'sound off' about inter-professional relations may, for some people, have been too good a chance to miss. Other, more timid souls may feel that it is disloyal to speak negatively about their colleagues to 'an outsider' and their account will perhaps have a rosier tint than their everyday reality might suggest. In making my selection of comments, it must be borne in mind that it is *my* selection and it is only part of the whole. I have tried to be as even-handed as possible and I have been particularly aware of the need not to misrepresent what these doctors and nurses have been saying.

### CHANGING SCENES

The research from which this book developed was carried out in late 1989 and 1990. Many things have changed within the National Health Service since then. Indeed, the rapidity of change is frightening to observe, and even more frightening to have to participate in. The picture of inter-professional relations which is given here is a snapshot in time. So many aspects are changing from nurse training to hospital trusts, from internal markets to general practitioners' budgets. Nevertheless, the areas of difficulty which have been identified are unlikely to disappear with any of these changes. The dynamics and factors influential in affecting how doctors and nurses work together are less changing and the need for conflict and differences of opinion remain.

The exploratory nature of the research meant that it made sense to develop theories as to cause and effect as the research progressed. There was no need of 'grand theory' when the investigations began, and it is of little use now. For those who do need the 'security blanket' of a theory, then the method use was that of 'grounded theory' (Glaser and Strauss, 1968), 'theory' grounded in the experiences of the individual respondents as they were recounted in the interviews. It has become apparent as the research developed that there were many factors influencing the experiences of the nurses and doctors we interviewed. Many of these have been identified but I am sure there are others which have been given insufficient attention. The arguments being presented here are tentative. Collingwood and Myers (1937) gave the following warning to historians but it is for all of us to heed:

'The conflicts are too complex the issues too obscure, the cross-currents too numerous the decisions too local to make possible the appreciation of any single formula to their solution: and is at least reassuring some times to remember that if we found such a formula we should unquestionably be wrong.'

# 2

# Common aims, contrasting cultures

'. . .it was a heated argument at full pace right in the middle of the ward and it was really, really bad. It was demoralising for us, for everybody. The patients cried, the ones who could understand what was going on, they were crying. I did the ward round afterwards because of the heated argument between the teams, so I had to intervene and carry on with the ward round, but I felt so bad for some time. It was not nice.' *Registrar*

This is not the sort of scene we expect to encounter in hospitals. We take it for granted that doctors and nurses work together, co-operating in looking after the patients. As patients we see the problems under which nurses and doctors have to function but we are perhaps less sensitive to the tensions within the health care team.

## GREAT EXPECTATIONS

As patients, and we are all likely to be patients sometime, we tend to be less critical of the service we gratefully receive at the hands of nurses and doctors compared with services we seek elsewhere. We are more likely to hear complaints about the behaviour of the police, or the inadequacies of social workers. We are not in the habit of listening to diatribes against the way in which doctors and nurses care for their patients. There may be complaints about conditions, buildings, and staffing levels and the occasional 'rotten apple' but it is relatively rare to hear criticisms of the people who do the caring in hospitals.

We feel we receive something special from nurses and doctors. We expect doctors and nurses to put the patient first and themselves second. We expect the doctor to come to our bedside in the middle of the night, whether inside or outside hospital. We expect doctors to know what is wrong with us and be able to do something about it. We expect nurses to wipe our bottoms, blow our noses, or clean up our vomit without frowning or complaining. We expect nurses to be smiling and friendly, listening to our worries and telling us 'it's alright', just as our mother might comfort us.

We are aghast when a nurse swears, we are dismayed when she is moody, we are mortified if she forgets our name. We are indignant if the doctor is offhand with us; we are perturbed if he doesn't remember what he said to us yesterday, we are angry if he can't find the time to talk to us.

These then are elements of our stereotypes and expectations: nurses are to be sweet-tempered and soothing, paying us particular and special attention. Doctors are to have the time and the inclination to talk to us. We expect them to care about us. More, perhaps than we care about them.

## Patient feelings

As patients, we are vulnerable. We have to trust those in whose care we have been placed. We must feel confident in the skills, secure in the attentions and reassured by the routines of the nurses and doctors. Also, we must be able to feel that each knows what the other is doing: that they are working as a team. Poor communication between those who are looking after us can result in catastrophes. There are countless apocryphal stories about the hospital. The hospital is a place that frightens us. It is a place in which we lose our autonomy and freedom of action. It is a place in which we give up our bodies to 'the professionals'.

The hospital is also a place in which we are 'the outsiders'. It is the health care workers who are 'the insiders', who work there all the time and know the system. The patients, who are unfamiliar with the system, the building, the rituals and language can feel particularly naked and vulnerable. For many of us, the hospital is a place of fear, associated with pain and with dying.

### The hospital's needs

Despite such feelings, the hospital has need of us. It needs its patients, who are 'imported' from outside, attended to and despatched, feet first or otherwise, from the hospital. The hospital 'borrows' our bodies for a while. Our bodies will be processed: monitored, tested, incised, dosed, irradiated. Some bodies will be tricky to deal with, others more straightforward. None of us will stay that long, not these days anyway. There is a faster and faster throughput, aided by medical research and technology. More and more of us are needed to lend our bodies for shorter and shorter periods of time.

The hospital's demand for us seems insatiable. It claims more and more territory, inventing new ways to adjust and repair our bodies when they reach ever greater stages of disrepair and decrepitude. The hospital's demand is so acute that preventing cannot be the focus of their attention, their main aim is the servicing of our illnesses and diseases. It is what keeps the hospital system going.

Despite this, it is not the hospital and all that it has to offer which has improved our life expectancy in this century (McKeown, 1976); those gains have been achieved through improvements in sanitation, housing and welfare provision rather than through health care. Rather, the hospital is the centre of what we see as being health care in Britain today. The hospital is the place where we are repaired, made whole again, returned to our normal lives; and for this we ought to be, and we are, grateful.

### WHY WORK IN HOSPITALS?

Why do people want to work in hospitals? What inspires a young person to choose to spend their working life looking after and working for the benefit of others in hospitals? What makes someone want to spend their life with people who are ill and diseased and whom the rest of us shun? A similar question poses itself about a prison officer who chooses to live their working life in prisons: an existence used as a punishment for others.

Patients sometimes are our modern-day lepers. Those who are in contact with our pariahs do what we cannot do and for this we attribute qualities such as bravery and self-sacrifice to them. In order to do such work one needs to have a sense of vocation, a notion that is strongly held within the ranks of nurses (Mackay, 1989, p.132 *passim*). There continues to be a sense of self-denial in nursing: a reflection of the continuing influence of the nuns and the importance of religion on the shape and values of nursing (Abel-Smith, 1960, Chapter 1). Why should nurses' vocation be directed towards caring for the sick in hospitals?

## The doctor's choice

Like us, doctors and nurses are likely to see the hospital as being **the** place in which the sick are cared for. For them, as for us, the hospital may be viewed with awe: it **is** something special that goes on there, something almost magical where pain can be removed and death defied. Perhaps those who choose to work in hospitals are particularly anxious to control and fight death.* Certainly those who make pronouncements on our bodies and state of health enjoy great power and authority. (For a discussion of the different types of authority enjoyed by medical practitioners, refer to Maclean, 1974. pp.78-80). The particular rituals and ceremonies of the hospital enhance the authority of doctors and the awe in which they are held.†

We seek doctors when we face situations with which we cannot deal ourselves. We call in the trouble-shooter, the warrior, the magician who will intervene or fight on our behalf. The adversary is death. It is a role which demands action. When the doctor can do nothing, it is the kiss of death for the patient. There is no hope now that the doctor has made his pronouncement. The doctor's magic cannot work, the adversary is too strong. Faced with a situation in which no useful action can be taken, the doctor loses some of his 'specialness' (Becker *et al.*, 1961). He has to abandon us. It is no accident that the specialties given the lowest status within the medical profession are those where there is little return for any 'action' which is taken.

---

\* A useful discussion of the motivations towards working in hospices with the dying is given by Vachon, 1978.
† Various aspects of these issues are discussed in: Goffman, 1969; Foucalt, 1973; Maclean, 1974; Wolf, 1986; Campbell-Heider and Pollock, 1987.

Nurses too, prefer the action specialties rather than those in which medical action is doomed to failure (Mackay, 1989, p.47; Melia, 1987, p.137). Medical science can do little for the permanently disabled, the mentally handicapped, the elderly and for them the doctor offers no hope. When medical science is powerless, doctors lose their interest. A reflection of that loss of interest is evident in the funding of specialties within the NHS: the worst funded are those furthest from the curative process (Davidson, 1987, p.8).

*Limitations*

Doctors are aware of the limits of medical science and they are aware of the limits of their training. They are frequently embarrassed by these limits. Yet the patient, so it seems, places inordinate faith in medicine. The doctor cannot disappoint, so he doesn't communicate. If contact with the patient is reduced, the possibility of this embarrassment, of the limits of medical science, will be minimised. Doctors have given their lives to medicine insofar as medicine is their career. They cannot therefore easily own to the inadequacies of medicine. So, for the doctor, the 'don't know' of uncertainty can soon become the 'I don't want to know' refusal to hear the patient.

As medical students, the promises of medical science and the benefits of action, have been inculcated. Their greatest dislike is feeling 'useless' (Firth, 1986, p.1179). With the action, there is the imagery of the conquering hero, the one with special powers to whom we are deeply grateful and respectful. The image of this life-saving hero may be particularly attractive to the intellectually gifted young person who is in a position to choose medicine.

## Occupational choice

Mackie (1967) has argued that if there is an unwelcome part of ourselves for which we cannot care, we may hope that others can care for that part of us. It may be that people who offer us care would like such care themselves. Menzies (1970, p.33) notes that there is a painful lack of support given to student nurses while they can see the care and attention given to patients. Some of the nurses who were interviewed mentioned this as one aspect influencing their choice of occupation. Others choose their occupation so that they will be needed by others, or that others are dependent on them. The reasons for occupational choice are extremely varied, as are the reasons why people remain in those occupations. Once they are part of the hospital, these carers are assured of being highly esteemed and respected by us, the outsiders.

This is not to deny that some patients are ungrateful and surly when they are in contact with hospitals. Particular indignation is reserved for those who are not suitably grateful for the services they receive in hospitals. The violent man in the accident and emergency department, and the grumpy woman in the medical ward, both reaffirm our respect for those who do the caring.

So it is with surprise that we greet disagreement and conflict among those who are looking after us. We do not expect doctors and nurses to be bickering about who is to do what, or what is the best course of action. To a great extent, as patients, we shall not have to become aware of any differences of opinion because they will be conducted quietly and out of our hearing. The presence of conflict is disguised in order to maintain our trust and confidence in the treatment we are receiving and the care we are being given. However, although appearances are maintained, they are only appearances. There is a substantial degree of conflict between nurses and doctors. This shouldn't really come as any surprise. It is incredibly difficult to work with other people and not have disagreements and differences of opinion. It is normal to have conflicts, and suspicious if there are none. What is perhaps surprising is that some doctors and nurses deny the presence of any conflict or even irritations. This denial is perhaps a reflection of the need of some in the hospital world to present a secure and harmonious environment to all its visitors.

It is remarkable that there is not even more conflict. Severe stress is involved in nursing and doctoring: actions often have to be decisive and sure, reactions fast, emotional strength great, and physical endurance substantial. Doctors and nurses have to deal with situations in which it is only too easy to panic, to make mistakes and to blame others. It is a difficult working situation to face each day with equanimity. It is doctors and nurses who are responsible for our well-being. There is pressure in that responsibility. It is an onerous burden which it is often difficult to carry.

## THE IMPORTANCE OF GOOD WORKING RELATIONSHIPS

It is hard to overstate the importance of 'good' working relationships in health care. As in any sphere of activity, things go wrong, accidents happen and mistakes are made. But in hospital, mistakes can be fatal. Because people's lives and their quality of life are potentially at risk, great care has to be taken at each and every level. The wrong diet, the wrong drug, the wrong tests, the wrong name and the wrong operation are potential hazards. The world of the hospital 'is a peculiarly unforgiving work environment' (Martin, 1984, p.235). And when something goes wrong, somebody is blamed and somebody has to be responsible. Taking care of patients is, therefore, burdensome.

The potential suffering of patients is one of the recurring themes that emerges from the interviews as to why good inter-professional relationships are so important. It is a theme which recurs frequently in the literature from the USA (Crowley and Wollner, 1987; Horsley, 1987; Schmitt and Williams, 1985). There are obvious risks to the patients when working relationships are not good. Warning about the importance of good working relationships has also been expressed with regard to hospitals in the UK (Martin, 1984).

'. . .last year, again it was the Senior Registrar, we had a tracheotomy patient, the tracheotomy tube was a problem in that it wasn't the right size, he was actually putting the patient's life at risk and nobody would listen to me. And that's when I phoned my Consultant when he was on holiday and he got things sorted out within an hour, and came back in and said "well, you were right all the time". . .'
*Sister*

'I think if you have got a doctor and a nurse that work together, you don't get confusing messages given to the patient about what is going to happen. If the nurse understands what the doctor is thinking you are not going to get two different things told to the patient and they will probably feel confident (because) of that.' *Senior House Officer*

'. . . the absence of good working relationships . . . is a recipe for catastrophe in patient care. . . .' *Professor*

'If you've got a happy ward relationship with a doctor, the rest of the staff are happy, the patients are happy, and they get better much quicker. If a patient can see a doctor and nurse relationship, you know, working well, it gives them more confidence in the nurse and the doctor.' *Sister*

'I was really cross last week when one of the Consultants I was saying something to on the ward about a patient and he said "Shhh!" I said "No, I am not going to shut-up!" If they try and shut me up about something that needs to be said about a patient or the way she is being managed – that's when I get really cross. . . . We had a patient who had been admitted under one team and they wanted her referred to another team and that team wouldn't accept her. It went on like this for about a week, well for five days and I felt the lady was really deteriorating and there was no-one being responsible for her, so that is what I was angry about.' *Sister*

## Reasons for conflict

There is often good reason for nurses or doctors to become angry with one another. Breakdowns of communication and failures of memory can seriously affect patients. It is not only 'the mechanics' of the system which can affect patient care, but the quality of the relationships between doctors and nurses. If doctors and nurses don't hear of the 'feelings' which one another have about a patient, if they are not aware of the frustrations being experienced by colleagues, then their decisions and actions will be taken without sufficient knowledge.

Similarly, if the members of a group are constantly changing it makes working together difficult. In hospitals doctors and nurses move around from ward to ward and specialty to specialty. The 'Cook's Tour' method of training favoured in both occupations ensures that familiar faces are soon replaced by strange faces. Pre-registration House Officers have only just settled in when they are moved on to get experience of another specialty; student nurses come and go just as quickly. In addition, although qualified nurses will spend longer in their posts, attempts to make a career in nursing often mean leaving one specialty and going into another (Appendix C). So when it's glibly stated that nurses and doctors ought to work as a team, given the movement of staff, it can be a lot easier said than done.

Doctors and nurses are not simply members of an occupational group. First and foremost, they are individuals and quite different from one another. It is easy to ignore the individual when discussing the group.

## DOCTORS' AND NURSES' – BACKGROUNDS AND CAREER CHOICES

### Familial connections

Traditionally there has been an acceptance that doctors come from backgrounds in which one or more members of the family are doctors. In the recent past, applicants to medical school have been looked on favourably if they had a parent who was a doctor (Johnson, 1971). Today, increasing emphasis is being made on academic qualifications and in some cases, candidates may not be interviewed, their 'paper' qualifications being enough (Young, 1981).

The majority of nurses and doctors do not have a nurse or a doctor in their (extended) family. Less than a third of doctors in the sample had a doctor in the family whether as parent, aunt or sibling, etc. (Appendix D).

This proportion is slightly lower than that found in other studies: Allen (1988) found that 42% of a sample of doctors had a medical connection in their family. A similar level of family influence was found in the USA (Becker *et al.*, 1961), 48% of the sample having relatives in medicine. Just over one third of the nurses said a member of their family had been, or still were, nurses.

## Career choices

Obviously, if there is a nurse or a doctor somewhere in the family, and it doesn't need to be the immediate family, the option or possibility of working in health care exists. Having a medical or nursing family background does exert some influence in choosing a career. However, only 16% of doctors and 17% of nurses interviewed mentioned the influence of family and friends in making their career choice (Appendix E). It seems that having a nurse or a doctor in the family is more of a disincentive than an incentive to take up either occupation.

### *Leaving the job*

Most nurses and doctors enter the job when they are young and although some will have worked in other fields, the majority will have little experience of other types of work. (It is perhaps surprising that 15% of doctors and 28% of nurses had previously embarked on or wanted to follow another career.) They commit themselves to their occupations by training for three years as nurses, and five years in medical school for doctors. For both it is a substantial investment in terms of time and energy. Yet surprisingly, over 50% of doctors and over 50% of nurses asked this question have considered leaving (Appendix F). For half of these, any thoughts of leaving had been general with no specific occupation in mind. However, the other half had considered specific occupations: drama school, personnel management, psychotherapy, corporate law, graphic art, vet, police, and many others. For some, thoughts of leaving are mere pipe-dreams, considered at times when their morale is at a particularly low point. Others are distinctly unhappy with the occupation they have chosen. This has been reported from other research. Allen (1988, p.291) reported that from an overall sample, 32% of female doctors and 27% of male doctors interviewed had regretted their career decision. The proportion for those doctors who had qualified in 1981 was much higher: 49% of females and 44% of males regretted their decision (Allen, 1988, p.296). However, it is not always easy to leave:

'That's why I haven't left!! I think I learned quite quickly that the grass is always greener on the other side. But speaking to people in other professions and other jobs it's quite clear that the frustrations in medicine are felt by everyone in every job. So, no I have not made any serious attempt of finding an alternative career.' *House Officer*

'Probably management. . .personnel management. I think that's what I would do if I gave up. . . I usually think it at five in the morning. . . . (laughs)' *Senior House Officer*

'I love my job but you know there are times when you're busy and just the way things are and you think about getting out, of the shift working and just. . . mostly the shift working, I think thats what it is. I'd love to get a Monday to Friday job and not work at weekends. But I can't do anything else, so. . . .! I came straight in from school.' *Staff Nurse*

'. . . when you discover the unreasonable things that are expected of you; when you discover how mundane a lot of the things you are asked to treat are; I think that a lot of people become very disillusioned with it. . .' *Senior House Officer*

The reason many do not leave is because they have invested so much in their training and work experience that they feel unable to 'throw it all away'. It is perhaps a poor reason for staying in a job, but the reason is likely to be given by members of many occupations. The non-transferability of skills from one job to another is a problem of any highly-specialized society. Job specific skills are so often sought by employers that the range and depth of experience in other fields is overlooked. It is a problem often encountered by women who have spent some time managing a household and child rearing. After all, what performance in any occupation could possibly be enhanced by having highly-honed time-management and prioritizing skills?

### Absenteeism

Within nursing there is a relatively high incidence of absenteeism. Going absent for a couple of days is one way in which nurses can cope with a less than satisfying work environment. Absenteeism can act as a safety valve for the stresses and frustrations experienced by nurses when they do not want, or are unable, to leave nursing (Mackay, 1989, p.59).

## Job dissatisfaction

The prevalence of thoughts about leaving nursing and medicine is, however, an indication of the dissatisfaction that nurses and doctors experience in their everyday work. Quite apart from the personal costs borne in terms of stress and frustration, there are costs to the health service. An over-worked and under-appreciated young nurse or doctor is unlikely to give high quality health care. Indeed, the idea of giving care to another when no-one seems to be caring for you, must surely produce resentment. Slogging out the battle against understaffing is an old refrain from nursing (Mackay, 1989, p.60). It means that nurses vote with their feet and leave the NHS. For junior doctors, the pressures and responsibilities of hospital work can ensure a speedy retreat to the calmer life of the general practitioner.

Even if the embattled young nurses and doctors can continue to deliver a reasonable standard of care, it will be at a personal cost which will also be borne by the health service when it results in a blasé and cynical workforce. In turn there will be a cost in patient care: 'the way we treat students and junior doctors is surely reflected in the way that they in turn treat their patients' (Blanche, 1988, p.160). In a few years, those doctors who survive their baptism by fire will superintend their own junior doctors, fresh from medical school. The demands made on the senior doctors when they were juniors are by this time fondly remembered and revisited on their juniors: 'it was good for us, it will be good for you', quite forgetting of course, that the 'advances' of technology and in particular 'the bleep' which cause today's junior doctors to have an unacceptably stressful and pressured worklife.

The particular frustrations and stresses of these doctors and nurses will be examined in later chapters. For the moment, however, it is enough to note that any exhortations to maximise inter-professional teamwork may ring hollow in the ears of those who are struggling to cope in the present conditions of the NHS.

Although there are similarities in the problems facing doctors and nurses caused by the present stringent economies in the health service, there are great disparities in the occupational worlds which each face. It is to these differences that attention must turn in order to fully appreciate the factors contributing to the irritations and difficulties experienced by members of the two groups. There are many differences between these two occupational groups, one an aspiring profession, the other a fully-established profession, which are often not given sufficient attention. Similarly, it is useful to examine some of the differences which affect the experiences of individuals **within** each occupation.

THE SITUATION IN SCOTLAND AND ENGLAND

One hundred and thirteen of the interviews took place in Scotland. There were not any outstanding differences, but there were subtle variations in the situations facing nurses and doctors in Scotland in comparison with England. As regards Health Authorities expenditure, in Scotland it is £423.35 per head of population, compared with £311.72 in England (Central Statistical Office 1992). There is also a general air of prosperity in the hospitals that were visited, which contrasted strikingly with the two district hospital locations in England.

Scotland has a small population which is widely dispersed in the north and south, with the central belt being much more densely populated. Scotland seems to have a more 'local' feel to it (although I may be biased); it is much easier for one Consultant to know and to have heard of a colleague elsewhere than it is in England. It may also be easier for Consultants to feel and to act as 'big fish' in such a relatively small pond.

### Differences in attitude

Scotland has traditionally been associated with according particular respect for education and those who are educated. The overall impression from the interviews in Scotland (with some notable exceptions) is that more deference is given by nurses towards members of the medical profession. There seems to be greater distance between nursing and medical staff in the Scottish teaching hospital compared with the London teaching hospital. Similarly, many of those interviewed felt that Scottish nurses were less assertive than their English counterparts.

At the same time it seems that the dominance of the 'nursing hierarchy' over nurses in the Scottish teaching hospital may be greater. According to a Nursing Officer in a Scottish teaching hospital, nursing 'is very much more disciplined in Scotland than it was in London'. At a national level, nursing in Scotland gives the impression of having been able to assert its rightful place alongside the medical profession to a greater extent than in England. In Scotland, nurses have retained the right to be represented at health board level, albeit only in an advisory capacity. Their English colleagues have not retained this right, their presence is discretionary (although at the moment it seems highly unlikely that nurses would actually be excluded). Women seem to have also held more places in senior positions within nursing in Scotland. In England more men appear to have attained senior positions in nursing, at least in the five locations visited.

Although there is little difference in the tasks that nurses do in Scotland and England, comments were made about the greater willingness of nurses in the Scottish teaching hospital to accompany doctors on their ward rounds than in, say, a London teaching hospital. (Differences in the approach taken to teaching medical students on the wards have been identified in Scotland and England (Atkinson, 1977.) This may have been a reflection of the hospitals in which the interviews were conducted: both tended to recruit nurses from the local, rather than the national, labour market. This could mean that because fewer nurses had had to leave home they had less wide experience that might produce a more questioning attitude to the status quo. In turn, the reliance on local nurses may result in other differences. Thus, 'there is definitely more class distinction up here I would think' (*Nursing Officer*).

The overall impression, therefore, in Scotland is that nurses at ward level are more deferential to doctors while, at the most senior level, nurses have been better able to resist moves to weaken their influence in management decisions than their English counterparts. The result is an apparently more hierarchical system in which greater deference and respect is given to the medical profession, and to senior nurses. Similarly, tensions between nursing and medicine can be expressed at senior levels allowing for a corresponding reduction in tension at ward level.

## TEACHING AND NON-TEACHING HOSPITALS

### Medical staff opinion

Substantial differences between teaching and non-teaching hospitals were felt to exist by the nurses and doctors who had worked in both. ('Teaching hospitals' are those hospitals to which a University Medical School is attached, or which places its students in, that hospital. Non-teaching hospitals do not routinely have medical students on the wards. Generally speaking, greater prestige is accorded to those nurses and doctors who work in teaching hospitals compared with those who work in non-teaching hospitals.) District hospitals were generally felt to be friendlier than teaching hospitals, with the result that nurses and doctors were likely to be more helpful to one another. This markedly affected working relationships:

'Here, although they are nice I still feel it is much more formal, whereas in [the District General Hospital] I found that the nurses were all on first name terms. Whereas here I still don't know all the nurses' names and it is very much you know Sister this and Sister that, and they tend to call me Doctor all the time.' *House Officer, Teaching Hospital*

'Like in the teaching hospitals, there are some and they come from there and you think "Oh my God" . . . "I can't stand them". . . [they're] snotty. Treat nurses like second class citizens.' *Staff Nurse, District General Hospital*

'I think Doctors' egos were bigger. I think because of that relationships were a bit more awkward and things got a bit heated, but that happens here as well. Yes, they were a bit different. It was a bit more formal and old-fashioned I think that is the right word.' *House Officer, District General Hospital*

'I think the Consultants at teaching hospitals are a lot

nastier. They have probably had to fight a lot harder to get where they are. The Consultants I had at the teaching hospital were out to get you really, whereas these ones are out to help you.' *House Officer, District General Hospital*

Thus, teaching hospitals were felt to be more formal, doctors more 'superior', nurses busier and less helpful to doctors. These comments refer to teaching hospitals in both Scotland and England. There is a general acceptance that if a doctor is going to establish a successful career then a post in a teaching hospital is highly desirable. There is a perceived trade-off between the 'easier' working relationships in the District General Hospital and the greater career prospects but more competitive atmosphere in teaching hospitals. In district hospitals, many junior doctors felt they gained wider experience than in teaching hospitals where there were greater numbers of doctors and competition for 'interesting' was cases more fierce. Also, the competitive jostling for places in teaching hospitals was one factor influencing junior doctors to move to non-teaching hospitals. It is not altogether surprising that junior House Officers have been found to experience greater stress in teaching hospitals compared to non-teaching hospitals (Firth-Cozens, 1987).

## Nursing staff opinion

Just as a difference is perceived in the attitude and behaviour of the medical staff between teaching and district hospitals, there are also differences within the ranks of nurses. The different social class of nurses in teaching hospitals, and in London teaching hospitals in particular, was mentioned quite often. It certainly appeared during the interviews that nurses' accents in teaching hospitals were likely to be less regionally identifiable than those of their colleagues working in district hospitals. Doctors and nurses were more likely to come from the same, or a similar, social class to doctors especially in the London teaching hospital. In recent research, it has been found that nurses in the south-east were more likely than other nurses to have considered becoming a doctor (Soothill and Bradby, 1992). It is worth noting that most nurses who reach the highest posts within nursing and associated bodies appear to have come from a teaching hospital background. In the past there has been a general acceptance that teaching hospitals were able to select the most highly qualified nurses because they were attached to a university medical school (Birch, 1975, p.18). An ex-nurse commented that it was well known in London hospitals that among the new student nurses 'some girls miss their mothers, while other girls miss their ponies'. The recent and increasing difficulty in recruiting nurses to London teaching hospitals has, however, meant that more reliance may now have to be placed on a local labour force. This may lead to a greater heterogeneity of nursing staff:

> 'I think that perhaps the best nurses I've come across have been in teaching hospitals. But also I think the worst nurses have also been in teaching hospitals. So I think you get two extremes.' *Consultant, London Teaching Hospital*

## London versus the Provinces

Differences also exist between teaching hospitals in London and those in the provinces. There is a certain *cachet* in training in a London teaching hospital but the greater formality, as for example in the professorial units with their 'Grand Rounds', may result in less willingness to adopt a student-friendly approach. Some of the provincial teaching hospitals have, for example, encouraged deferred entry of medical students so that they can have a break between school and university. Deferred entry is positively discouraged at some, and barely tolerated at other, London teaching hospitals. Obviously, breadth of external experience is not always seen as helpful for potential members of the future elite of the medical profession.

## RECRUITMENT AND CLASS

Despite a widening of the group from which doctors are recruited, they continue to be drawn from a relatively narrow section of society. However, nurses, like secretaries, are drawn 'from a broad spectrum of social backgrounds' (Robinson, 1989, p.162; Stacey, 1988a, p.189). There have been substantial class divisions within nursing since the times of Florence Nightingale (Bellaby and Oribabor, 1980, p.170). Traditionally it has been the case within nursing that upper class women have directed the activities of lower class women. The matrons of yesterday, the 'lady superintendents', were 'superior' women who could quite easily frighten doctors. As one Consultant reminisced:

> 'When I was a House Surgeon I remember the first day on a job running along one surgical corridor, around a corner and not quite bumping into the Matron. It was just as well for me because in those days the matron was a big girl and I was much less than I am now. But I remember her saying to me 'oh Doctor, you must never run in a hospital you know, unless in the event of fire and haemorrhage you know. That means you are personally haemorrhaging or you are personally on fire.' *Consultant*

## Class divisions

These Matrons of yesterday were doughty women whose path was not crossed lightly. They defended their nurses and they ruled them with a rod of iron. The military discipline so beloved within nursing was a way of keeping the lower orders of nurses in their place. The strong emphasis on discipline within nursing continues, but is increasingly becoming dysfunctional. As mentioned above, there still seems to be some evidence of a class division within the ranks of nurses, at least in teaching hospitals. It is unclear to what extent there are class divisions within the ranks of nurses in non-teaching hospitals or teaching hospitals outside London.

The presence of a class division within nursing is often obscured. Nursing it seems is more concerned with the encroachments of men into the senior positions at local and national level (Carpenter, 1977, p.180) than with its internal divisions. The men who are rising within nursing are often from lower class backgrounds than the females they have replaced (Carpenter, 1977). It is possible that the recent reverses suffered by nursing at the top levels within hospitals are related to the diminishing numbers of upper class women within nursing.

### Effects of social class

The social class of each nurse will exert some influence on their relationships with doctors. The Sister who is married to a Consultant is likely to have her views attended to. The Sister who is married to a postman will perhaps have to rely more heavily on personal qualities and skills in the job if she is to gain equal attention. We are highly tuned to the personal cues given by accents and demeanour, and these are bound to affect our working relationships. In a similar way, the local nurse who has never left the area is likely to have a quite different relationship with doctors compared with the nurse who has trained elsewhere and has travelled. (The easier relationships reported by the nurses who had trained overseas in part reflects the influence of the class system on doctor–nurse interactions.) It is only when doctors are unfamiliar with the nurses that they see the uniform rather than the person wearing it. Once personal contact has been established, the various signals as to class and background will be communicated. When doctors refer to the great variations between nurses, they are implicitly referring to aspects of class as well as competence. There is little doubt that the inter-professional relationships of nurses will reflect the influence of different social and class backgrounds.

### Effects of training overseas

Doctors who have undertaken their medical training in other countries may find themselves unaffected by the class system, as is the case with the few nurses in the sample who had trained overseas. Relationships between nurses and overseas-trained doctors may be less formal. There may be differences in the style of communication and in expectations regarding what tasks nurses can and cannot do. However, doctors who have trained overseas may encounter discrimination. This is particularly likely to be the case for those who have trained in Africa, the Indian sub-continent and in the Middle East. Research has shown that these doctors experience discrimination in employment (Community Relations Commission, 1976; Smith, 1980). They will also experience discrimination in the way they are treated by colleagues, both nurses and doctors. Many of the overseas doctors interviewed were from the higher stratas, of caste or class within their own society. For some of these doctors from Africa, India, and the Muslim world it was difficult to treat patients as anything but inferior. Similarly, it was not easy for some of these doctors to consider women as equals or worthy of respect – although the same can also be said about some of the homegrown doctors! Cultural differences are compounded by those of religion and social background. Overseas doctors' accounts of their relationships with nurses and doctors are likely to reflect the influence of these factors.

## SPECIALTIES

The experiences of nurses and doctors will vary considerably from one specialty to another. Working conditions and relations in an operating theatre are quite different from those in a psychiatric ward. Different lengths and types of training and preparation are required in different specialties. The length of patient stay, the average age of the patients, the seriousness of the medical condition, whether the condition is chronic or acute, the grade of junior doctor, the presence of a doctor, ward layout and size are some of the factors which also vary from specialty to specialty.

### Intensive Therapy Unit

An intensive therapy unit usually has a one to one, nurse-patient ratio. Patients in ITU are not normally there for a great length of time but they will be intensively nursed. Every little task has to be done for each patient giving a special intimacy with patients who may not be conscious. Nurses in ITU are highly trained with wide-ranging technical skills required to monitor the increasingly complex machinery and life-support systems. There are many patients who do not survive. This, and the particularly close attention that needs to be paid to each patient, ensures that ITU nursing is very stressful. The knowledge of the nurses is usually compared favourably with that of the medical staff, with the comments of ITU nurses being closely attended to, at least by the anaesthetists who work there, if not by the visiting doctors from other specialties. A doctor is often to be found in ITU and it is a specialty in which working relationships are felt to be particularly close. This closeness may be fostered by the acceptance of both nurses and doctors of a 'medical' model of care (Owens and Glennerster, 1990, p.1530).

## Care of the elderly

In medicine for the elderly, on the other hand, doctors are likely to be present less often. The length of stay for patients tends to be longer than in other specialties. There is little reliance on technology, the patients being in greater need of nursing care than medical intervention. Working with the elderly does not enjoy great status within the hospital pecking order, which means that the less able (or the less favoured) may find a post there which would be denied to them in another specialty. Of course, many nurses make a positive choice to work with the elderly and find particular rewards in caring for older patients. It is a specialty in which the traditional nursing skills of caring and support can be fully expressed. Nevertheless, for many nurses and doctors, caring for the elderly is not a favoured specialty. It is not a coincidence that overseas doctors and women doctors are often to be found in geriatric medicine units. It seems overseas doctors occupy positions in specialties that homegrown doctors do not want (Bradshaw, 1978). It has been argued that overseas doctors are often to be found in the 'wrong' specialties, that is, in specialties such as psychiatry and the care of the elderly where a knowledge of the local culture is particularly necessary (Smith, 1980, p.197). Among nurses there appears to be a division between those who have enthusiastically chosen to work with the elderly and those who have ended up there, having lost their enthusiasm for nursing altogether.

Nursing the elderly can be particularly difficult in the demands made on patience and physical stamina. People who are doubly incontinent are not usually the most sought-after patients. Training specific to caring for the elderly is not a requisite for working there. Doctors planning to move into general practice will be given experience of a range of specialties, including a few month's experience in medicine for the elderly. It is not universally enjoyed by the GP trainees who find the pace slow after, say, the adrenalin-producing experience in surgical specialties. The personality of the Sister in wards for the elderly seems to be particularly important if a 'good' ward atmosphere is to be achieved.

## General medical and surgical care

It is in the general medical and surgical wards that the pre-registration House Officers are to be found. It is here that the worrying first few months of doctoring are experienced: when confidence can be both undermined and/or established. In the general surgical and medical wards there are substantial differences in the way the ward 'feels'. There is still a slower pace to be found in medical compared with surgical wards. Heavily dependent patients requiring a great deal of nursing attention are often to be found in medical wards. Many patients will have been admitted as emergencies with heart and chest complaints. Patients will be admitted 'for investigation'. There may be certainty about the ailments of some patients and how they are best to be treated. For others there needs to be a wait-and-see approach while various tests are carried out, or differing drug regimens are tried and evaluated. There is, however, need for prompt action in medical wards dealing, for example, with coronary care or asthmatic patients.

Medical wards can be experienced as less exciting than surgical wards, where definite action in the form of surgery is taken. On the surgical ward there are admitting days and operating days in which the ward is all-a-bustle. New patients are being settled in to the ways of the ward while others are being despatched to theatre. There is lots to be done, lots to remember, the pace is fast. Patient throughput is speedy and there is hardly time to get to know the patients. But there is the feeling of accomplishing something: of getting lots of people in and out. You can often see a beginning, a middle and an end in surgical wards. The patient doesn't linger and there is relatively little uncertainty to tolerate. In the medical ward, uncertainty is usual and more difficult to cope with. The throughput can be slower and the patient contact greater, so that nurses and doctors will get to know their patients and their problems.

## Otolaryngology

Otolaryngology wards deal primarily with very short stay patients: tonsils, tooth extractions, adenoids, grommets are some of the bread and butter operations. There are, of course, some extremely serious cases to be found here, as in most specialties, where the prognosis of the patient is poor and length of patient stay correspondingly longer. But for the most part, the ear, nose and throat ward is a cheery ward with quite a bit of noise where the majority patients do not feel too poorly. The throughput of patients is fast and, as in general surgical wards, there is a feeling of getting on with the job and getting through the lists of patients for theatre.

## Operating theatres

Working in operating theatres is different from anywhere else in the hospital. The theatres are normally in a self-contained area, geographically isolated from the wards. They have their own common rooms and facilities. They are separate from the rest of the hospital. It is a place of great ritual and great informality. There is a shared intimacy between medical and nursing staff which is seldom experienced on the wards. Nurses and doctors are able to watch exactly what the other is doing. There is little leeway for sloppy practices. Exactness and precision are required from all in theatre. Handing the instruments to the surgeon, make incisions, suturing, counting swabs cannot be hit-and-miss affairs. The preferred ways of working of each surgeon are learned by the nursing staff. The personality and approach of each theatre Sister will be appreciated by each surgeon. In theatre, patients become 'cases'. There is the need to maintain some distance between the humanity of the patient and the enormity of making a substantial cut into that body. The gallows humour long-associated with theatre is a useful defence against the awesome fact of cutting into people every day. It is in theatre that medicine takes on its most dramatic form. That drama is denied in the children's wards.

## Paediatric care

In the paediatric wards, the atmosphere is quite different from the adults' wards. The decor will be brighter, there will be many pictures on the walls, toys and books dotted around and nurses in colourful aprons rather than the traditional nurses' uniforms. First names among the staff are usual here, and there is an emphasis on informality and not frightening the children. Procedures such as taking a blood sample will be carried out in the side rooms so that the other children do not have to hear or watch.

There will be a wide range of medical conditions among the children in the paediatric unit; there will be some with broken legs and there will be some with leukaemia. The attempt is always to make the atmosphere as light-hearted as possible, but the children's ward can bring the special distress of a dying child. And when a child has been a regular patient on the ward, visiting intermittently for treatment over the months, even years, it is not always easy to see the death as a welcome release. Doctors and nurses in paediatrics cannot stand on their dignity for too long; children have a way of pricking egos and not being respectors of status.

## Mental care

Wards dealing with the mentally ill and disturbed are also not great respectors of status. Both the medical and nursing staff tend to be more relaxed in psychiatry than other adult specialties. First name terms are common, as in paediatrics. There will be few nurses wearing uniform and there will be, at least in these hospitals, an attempt to disguise the custodial nature of some patients' stay. Patients in psychiatric wards can be extremely difficult to deal with: unpredictable, sometimes violent, extremely emotional or unemotional. No two patients are the same in psychiatry.

There is not a quick throughput. Time needs to be taken to establish trust and build up relationships with patients. There are few medical procedures necessary but there is a stronger emphasis on drugs. Psychiatry has long been the specialty in which male nurses are most likely to be found. There are also a relatively large number of female doctors. In psychiatry, there is likely to be a greater blurring of the roles of nurse and doctor and patient.

## Personalities and specialties

It is thought that different personality 'types' are attracted to particular specialties. There are a variety of stereotypes alive and well in hospitals regarding the personality 'types' in different specialties. The evidence suggests that the stereotypes of medical students, for example, do not change greatly during their years in medical school: 'either the stereotypes were impervious to reality of else they reflected it' (Harris, 1981, p.1677). Surgeons are 'prima donnas' who are doers rather than thinkers; physicians are chess players, while surgeons are rugby players. 'Orthapaedic surgeons – twice as strong as an ox, and half the brains', is the quote that goes along with them (*House Officer, Medicine*). 'Short people go for paediatrics!' (*House Officer, Medicine*). Kinder comments come regarding one's own specialty: 'psychiatrists can tolerate ambiguity' (*Psychiatrist*); 'cardiologists are more caring' (*Staff Nurse, Coronary Care*); 'radiotherapists are more relaxed' (*Charge Nurse, Medicine*); 'anaesthetists are friendlier' (*Senior House Officer, Anaesthetics*).

### Positive stereotypes

The positive stereotypes listed above may have some basis in fact. It has been shown, for example, from a sample of anaesthetists that they display particular personal characteristics not found in other medical practitioners (Reeve, 1980). There also appears to be differences in political outlook and medical philosophy between some specialties (Wakeford and Allery, 1986, p.1026). However, there is a 'chicken and egg' argument here: do people with particular personalities choose one specialty or does experience in a specialty emphasize certain personality features? Whatever the answer there are certainly many stereotypes informing to a greater or lesser degree people's attitudes and responses to colleagues in other specialties (Furnham *et al.*, 1981; Furnham, 1986).

Stereotypes can be particularly influential in the case of surgery with its image of the 'macho' surgeon. Women have been almost totally excluded from surgery and are grossly under-represented in FRCS results (Dowie, 1987). Such exclusion can have a long-term effect: 'It is evident that any growth in numbers of women Consultants is only likely in those specialties where women are already comparatively well represented at more junior levels' (Lawrence, 1987, p.139). There were no women in surgery above Junior House Officer level in the sample.

### Negative stereotypes

Negative stereotypes regarding particular specialties affect not only the status and prestige of medical and nursing staff but also that of patients. For example, Tuckett (1976, p.380) notes that mental patients seem to need cheaper food than patients in other specialties. Similarly, in the recent past, the distribution of funding within the NHS has been to favour the high-intervention acute specialties at the expense of the low-intervention chronic specialties such as medicine for the elderly, mental handicap and mental illness (Davidson, 1987, p.7; Batchelor, 1984, p.74). Also, as noted earlier, it is an orientation which many nurses also share, many of whom express a preference for the high-intervention specialties.

In addition, there are likely to be more unregistered nurses working in mental handicap and care of the elderly (Owens and Glennerster, 1990, p.36). These same specialties are likely to be less often visited by medical staff, a situation which potentially leads to trouble regarding the quality of patient care (Martin, 1984, p.81).

Each specialty has its own character and specialties were chosen with particular care in order to allow for some of the differences mentioned above which contribute to this character. This must be borne in mind when considering the experiences recounted throughout the book.

There are also extremely specialised units, some so specialized that there may be only one such unit in each health authority region. Such a specialism might be a cardio-thoracic unit, or a centre for burns and plastic surgery. Teaching hospitals are likely to have a greater range of specialties than district hospitals. Teaching hospitals are also likely to have more 'interesting' or unusual cases sent to them by their district hospital colleagues. In turn, this adds to the prestige and status of the teaching hospital and its medical and nursing staff. However, this may also produce additional pressure for staff as they attempt to meet the often conflicting needs of residents from their own district and referrals from other districts.

THE DIFFERENT GRADES

The grade of the nurse and the doctor will substantially affect their experience and perception of inter-professional relations. Each grade experiences different priorities and pressures. The Staff Nurse has differing concerns from the Consultant, as does the newly-appointed House Officer in comparison with the Senior Registrar.

**Doctors**

*Junior House Officers*

Junior House Officers are newly-qualified doctors who spend their first year gaining experience in the general surgical and medical wards. There are few mature House Officers, most are in their early 20s. They are on the bottom rung of the hierarchy of the medical 'team'. They have to perform well for their Consultant in order to get their passport to a successful career, a good reference, from their Consultant. They are in the process of learning how to please their seniors. Their mentors will be the Senior House Officers (and in their absence the Registrars), who will advise them on the preferences of the Consultant and Senior Registrar. In reality, the new House Officer relies heavily on the Sisters and Staff Nurses for advice.

It is these House Officers who suffer the rigours of being on-call for unbelievably long hours and who must ensure that all is ready for the ward rounds of both the Consultant and Registrar. They have to work particularly closely with the nursing staff if they are to do their job effectively. They must have stamina to survive that first year, and some do not survive. Once they have completed their pre-registration year they become registered doctors and independent practitioners, and ready to take up a Senior House Officer post.

### Senior House Officers

The Senior House Officers who will have been qualified for at least a year are to be found in every specialty. They may as yet be undecided as to whether they wish to stay in hospital medicine or become general practitioners. They are not locked into any one specialty at this stage, they can move around, finding out the area of medicine to which they feel they are most suited. Some Senior House Officers will be working in a variety of specialties such as paediatrics, medicine for the elderly and psychiatry in a planned rota of experience as part of their GP training. Most importantly, these GP trainees are not dependent on the reference they receive from the Consultant. Relatively less power is, therefore, exerted on the doctor who wishes to move out of the hospital. All Senior House Officers will have to be on call, and in those specialties in which there are no Junior House Officers, that on-call duty is likely to be particularly onerous. Yet, Senior House Officers in psychiatry are less likely to be called than their colleagues in surgical wards.

Those Senior House Officers who have decided to stay in hospitals will have to work in their chosen specialty for a couple of years before they have a chance of being appointed to a Registrar's post. The references they receive from their seniors are particularly important. These are not simply written references but off-the-record telephone calls by which a Consultant can put in a quiet word for one of his juniors. It is in this process, when less effort is made on her behalf, that the female doctor may find out if her Consultant is less than enthusiastic about women in senior positions. It is the all-important informal network from which women tend to be excluded in medicine (Spencer and Podmore, 1987, p.2).

### Registrars

Doctors at Registrar grade are usually trying to pursue a career within hospital medicine. However, there are relatively few Consultants' posts available each year and many Registrars after a few years at this grade decide to move out of hospital medicine. It is a difficult and tension-filled time in which suitability for a hospital career is being established. Much time is spent trying to find a place where one might be appointed to, or groomed for, a Consultant's post. Doctors at Registrar level may remain in this grade for a number of years. The Registrar is less often on call than are Senior House Officers, but would be called when there is a problem which his juniors cannot resolve. It is also the Registrar (or Senior Registrar) who will call the Consultant out if necessary: a decision which is not to be taken lightly!

Once a Registrar's post has been obtained it is usually necessary to remain at that grade for two to four years. Promotion from this grade may be particularly difficult; in a 1984 census of doctors, 16% of Registrars were time-expired, i.e. it was four years or more since they entered that grade (Dowie, 1987, p.321).

There is a tremendous difference between specialties at Registrar grade. A surgical Registrar may wait a full five years to get a Senior Registrar post, while a psychiatric Senior Registrar may have to wait only three years for a Consultant's post. The Registrar who is to achieve a Consultant's post must first please his own Consultant, since, as the rungs of the ladder are mounted, the (informal) reference gains greater and greater importance. Throughout the years spent at this grade, the doctor continues to study in order to obtain membership of the one of the Royal Colleges, adding further pressure to those experienced in their normal working days.

### Senior Registrars

Senior Registrar posts are essentially 'waiting in the wings' posts where the doctor is virtually assured of becoming a Consultant, in time. It is an interim grade in which the uncertainty of Registrars, as to whether they will ever make it to a Consultant's post, is relatively absent. These are the doctors who are being groomed for teaching hospital Consultants' appointment and they are unlikely to be in their post for too many years before the prized post is achieved. Senior Registrars waiting for a Consultant's post keep things 'ticking-over' and running smoothly on the ward. They know exactly what their Consultants like and dislike, and act as trouble-shooters, sorting out difficulties and squabbles between junior doctors and nurses.

## Consultants

The Consultant leads the team of doctors, from pre-registration House Officer up to Senior Registrar grade. They are the top of the pile. It is the Consultant who has the final responsibility for patient care and who takes the blame when things go wrong. Compared with his district hospital colleagues, the teaching hospital Consultant is very seldom called out.

Consultants enjoy considerable independence and freedom of action. Once appointed they are likely to remain in post for 25 to 30 years. There is some difference in prestige between the Consultant working in a teaching hospital and the Consultant working in a district hospital. The former is based in a metropolitan area, and will normally have to undertake the teaching of medical students, hence the practice of Grand Rounds of the ward. Teaching hospitals Consultants also have an academic commitment and will need to maintain a research programme in order to enhance their own prestige and that of their department, as well as that of the hospital. Finally, teaching hospital Consultants have greater opportunities for undertaking private practice due to the combination of working in large metropolitan areas and having referrals from regional centres to national centres of medical excellence.

## Responsibilities and roles

Each level of doctor has differing levels of responsibility and a different role to play. All grades below Senior Registrar are 'training' grades. It takes many years to become a Consultant and doctors' 'training' lasts an inordinately long time; the rewards of a Consultant's post are great. The responsibilities and burdens of the post can also be substantial. Nevertheless, medicine is highly competitive and many sacrifices have to be made by those doctors wishing to climb the medical ladder. At each level doctors need to adjust their view of medicine and by the time they reach the coveted Consultant's post, they are extremely familiar with the politics of hospitals and the expectations which others may have of them.

## Nurses

On the nursing side there are two levels of registered nurses working at ward level: Staff Nurses and Sisters.

### Staff Nurses

Staff nurses have undertaken three years of training and are registered with the Royal College of Nursing. Staff Nurses are to be found in every hospital specialty. Promotion prospects vary from specialty to specialty and fairly rapid advance is possible in the less-favoured specialties. It is the Staff Nurse who will supervise the 'drug rounds' and oversee the activities of the junior and unqualified nursing staff. (There are still Enrolled Nurses to be found on the wards but as a grade they are being phased out. They are called Enrolled Nurses because their names are placed on the Roll of the Royal College of Nursing rather than on the Register. They are no longer being trained and Enrolled Nurses can 'convert' to Registered Nurses by undertaking further training.) Staff nurses have a substantial role in helping to train student nurses.

Staff nurses have relatively few 'basic' nursing tasks to do. Routine tasks such as bed baths and helping patients to get dressed will tend to be done by the student nurses and nursing auxiliaries. (Nursing auxiliaries, or nursing assistants as they are called in mental illness hospitals, carry out a substantial amount of 'nursing' work. That is, they are much concerned with the day-to-day welfare of patients and will spend a larger proportion of their day with the patients than will qualified nurses. They are often women of more mature years and tend to stay on one ward for a few years. Their contribution to patient care is often overlooked or at least not sufficiently credited.) Considerable responsibility falls on the shoulders of Staff Nurses. Since Sisters are often absent from the ward attending meetings, Staff Nurses have to 'act-up' and perform the duties of the Sister in her absence from the ward. As the 'nurse-in-charge', she will accompany the Consultant on his rounds and must be familiar with the up-to-date information on each patient.

Immediately after qualifying, Staff Nurses may move from one specialty to another, finding out – like Senior House Officers – in which specialty they would prefer to work. She may wish to undertake a specialist training course, for which competition is becoming keener, though when this has been completed, the Staff Nurse is less mobile. However, should she move to an area where that specialist skill is not used, she will likely suffer a drop in pay. For promotion, Staff Nurses – like doctors – depend on good reports of their work from their seniors.

### Sisters

Sisters, and their male equivalent of Charge Nurses are likely to have been qualified for at least three years (unless they are working in a specialty which has a particularly acute shortage of nurses or they are particularly gifted). When first appointed to Sister level they will be Junior Sisters, working under the overall guidance of a Senior Sister. Sisters enjoy a considerable amount of power over the junior nursing staff as well as the nursing auxiliaries and assistants. Their primary concern is with the smooth and efficient running of the ward and ensuring that standards of patient care are maintained. They are likely to remain in the post for a number of years. Junior Sisters may have to move wards in order to get a Senior Sister's grading. As a Senior Sister, promotion means moving from the clinical area into management. Some Senior Sisters resist all attempts to promote them out of the ward situation.

It is easy to talk about 'doctors' and 'nurses' yet it can be completely misleading. Each grade and level of nurse and doctor has different concerns and priorities. Within different specialties, the individual experiences and varying perceptions of the work all combine to make each individual quite distinctive. In talking in grand terms about 'nurses' and 'doctors' the great variety of situations and factors affecting each individual must be borne in mind.

# 3

# Different worlds

The phrase 'doctors and nurses' trips off the tongue. It is a phrase so commonly used that it is easy to overlook the different worlds and circumstances in which the members of each occupation exist. When the differences are considered, the difficulty involved in establishing any sort of 'equal' relationship between the two is obvious. Their worlds are so dissimilar that it is surprising that so much common ground has been established in day-to-day working relationships.

There are differences in the education and training of doctors and nurses. The entry requirements for medical training and nurse training are different. Intending doctors need to have at least three 'A' levels at Grade C or above, whereas nurses need to have a minimum of five GCSEs Grade C or above in England, or a minimum of 5 passes (band A, B or C) of the Scottish Certificate of Education examination (or equivalent) in Scotland. It appears that one-tenth of entrants to nursing have two or more A levels. (Strong and Robinson, 1988, p.159).

## Training schemes: medical versus nursing

Medical students spend five years in training, and nurses three years. Medical students are trained in universities, whereas nurses have until recently been trained in Schools of Nursing. (The introduction of the recommendations of Project 2000 has brought with it a change in location of nurse education. Nurses are now to be based in colleges or polytechnics.) In Schools of Nursing, which were linked to a group of hospitals, nurses were trained within an insulated and self-contained milieu. However, when nursing students also 'live in' the residences attached to the School of Nursing, the cloistered and claustrophobic atmosphere to which recruits to nursing have been subjected becomes evident. In contrast, although medical students share universities with a range of other undergraduates, it appears that relatively little interaction with non-medical students takes place. Participation in the 'broader' environment which education in the tertiary sector can provide may not always take place. Medical students appear to be isolated from and isolate themselves from the mainstream of the student population (Robson, 1973, p.415; McCormick, 1979, p.144). Nevertheless, until recently, it has been the case that nurses have been trained within the NHS, whereas doctors train within the higher education sector.

*Nursing training*

Nurse training has received substantial criticism over the years. The implementation of the Project 2000 recommendations means that nurse training will change and move into the realms of higher education. In the past, nurse training has been 'service-based', and although Project 2000 will mean that student nurses are no longer to be counted in the staffing levels on any ward, the greatest part of their training will continue to take place 'on the job'. The influence of practitioners will be reduced but not substantially. The nurse is still being trained to 'fit into' a system which is often antagonistic to academic knowledge, which extols the virtues of practice, and may be less than receptive to the new recruits. The nurse of old was cloistered in her school of nursing, nurses' residence and the hospital. There was little opportunity to explore or even become aware of alternative perspectives. Indoctrinated into the received wisdom of nursing, there was little opportunity to exercise independence in thought or action. Narrowly trained for a narrow existence, no questioning of the system or any part of it was to be fostered. A biddable and quiescent workforce was produced to service others: patients and doctors.

While nurses' training has been and remains predominantly practice-based, doctors' training places substantial emphasis on the theoretical and scientific components of medical knowledge. Although science may be a preferred subject for an applicant to study nursing, science is **the** required subject for the intending medical student. Indeed, for many doctors (and especially those in hospital medicine), medicine **is** science and doctors are seen to be, above all else, scientists. The lure of the scientific element in medicine was mentioned by 15% of the doctors as one of their reasons for choosing medicine (refer to Appendix E).

While there are some within the policy-making circles of nursing who seek to assert or establish a 'scientific' base for nursing practice, there is an accepted practical base to nursing. Nursing, in other words, is a practical skill rather than a skill based on theory and science. Within the ranks of nurses there is a decided anti-intellectual and anti-academic perspective (Bradshaw, 1984, p.11; Mackay, 1989, p.151 *passim*). Whether, or the extent to which, nursing can claim to have a scientific base is a debate beyond the scope of this book. However, the lack of a scientific and theoretical basis is one of the charges laid against nursing by some members of the medical profession.

### Medical training

Medical students in their training spend their first two years in a university setting, with forays into the clinical world taking place on a regular basis in the last three years. It is at this time that students gain some first-hand knowledge of a vast array of specialties: knowledge which will help inform their own career decisions. Many criticisms of medical training have been made. For example, Ellis (1988, p.138) has commented on 'its heavy emphasis on factual knowledge, even though much of this knowledge will be rapidly outdated.' Medical training with its scientific emphasis results unwittingly in less concern for patients (McCormick, 1979, p.24; Young, 1981). In particular, medical training has been criticized as being combative and through which doctors come to see colleagues as rivals and competitors (Pigache, 1991, p.29). Within medicine there is 'survival of the fittest rather than the best' doctors (Payne and Firth-Cozens, 1987, p.20), with the competitiveness seen by some medical students as being both destructive and an effective barrier to learning (Blanche, 1988, p.156).

Students normally enter medical training direct from school. They have little or no experience of other work or of the world outside. As nurses have been cloistered in their training, so intending doctors have been cloistered at school and then in their medical school training, with the constant need to study for and pass exams. The tunnel vision which can result (Brazell, 1987, p.96). means that doctors can fail to see beyond their own lives and world. Lacking experience of the struggles which others may face, in effect they have less chance to learn any respect or humility for others. As students or as doctors, they are not involved with or engaged with the 'common herd'. Doctors may pronounce judgements and care for their patients, but they may simultaneously be insulated from the reality of their patients' lives. They will be shocked by the lack of patients' knowledge about their bodies and they will shy away from their 'ignorant' patients' silly fears (Heiberg, 1987, pp.1602–3). They may fail to develop any compassion.

'Doctors. . . will remember that their first patient was an embalmed corpse. Much that bedevils the relationship between doctors and patients today can be traced back to a yearning by doctors to recover this lost, undemanding, and in this sense, ideal relationship.' *Marinker, 1974, p.452*

Too easily can the doctor become a 'body technician' with the narrow focus of medical training. The curriculum for medical students is already crammed and there is little time or opportunity to look beyond the medical school. It is no wonder that medical students 'tend to increase in cynicism and decrease in humanitarianism during their medical school experience' (Rezler, 1974, p.1023). The knock-on effects of these factors has been an over-emphasis within medicine on the academic and scientific aspects at the expense of the *art* of medicine, which is centrally concerned with patients and the ability of doctors to communicate with them (Parkhouse, 1991, p.291).

### Training objectives

While medical training can be seen as a 'toughening up' process preparing students for the rigours of a doctor's life, nurse training is an object lesson in submission. In nurse training, **others** get tough. The nurse is taught to follow rules, to be deferential to doctors, and the importance of routine is emphasized (Davies, cited in Kerrison, 1990, p.21). Nurse training 'advocated submission to those in authority both in nursing and medicine' (Mills, 1983, p.10).*

The competitiveness of medicine becomes apparent during the training. Doctors quickly learn to look after themselves. The independence on which doctors pride themselves and base their clinical judgement is reinforced by the competitive spirit necessary to survive in medicine. With no effort, doctors can adopt a superiority which ignores, or is blind to, the needs of others. This is a curious response to seek to evoke from those who have chosen a profession concerned with helping to heal others.

### Clinical experience

Substantial importance is accorded to the clinical experience within medicine. For this reason, even the most senior doctors within the medical profession pride themselves on, and continue to seek, involvement in clinical practice. Those nurses, however, seeking to advance to senior levels within nursing have to leave the clinical area. This fact is continually bemoaned and ridiculed by members of the medical profession.

'There is this pressure on nurses, ward nurses especially, ward sisters – if they're any good, to be promoted to become an administrative officer of some sort and it seems to me to be ridiculous that just as someone is getting good at their job in running the ward and the ward running like clockwork, they get pushed up into nurse management. . .' *Consultant*

'I have my reservations against that system of nursing officers, I think that they should be taking some nursing duties to keep in touch and always have a feel for how to nurse, and the day-to-day problems. Because if they sit in their offices for a long time they become detached.' *Registrar*

---

*   Detailed descriptions of the dynamics of nurse training are given by Birch, 1975; Melia, 1987; Mackay, 1989.

The lack of clinical involvement means that the most senior nurses are seen to lose touch with the practice of nursing. It also implicitly demonstrates if not a disdain, then the irrelevance of nursing practice for those nurses involved in managerial (or non-clinical) roles within the hospital. In this way, there is a stark contrast between the medical profession, which highly values clinical practice, and the nursing profession, which does not.

Tied in with medicine's 'scientific orientation' is the medical profession's preference for those specialties in which 'cures' can be effected. Nurses are only peripherally involved in the 'curing' of patients, in the diagnosis and prescriptions and treatments. Nurses are however, centrally involved in the caring which patients require: comfort-giving, physical caring and emotionally supporting aspects of health care. Nurses' labour is often emotional labour (James, 1989). It is an attention to, and care for, the patient's mental well-being which is not fostered in medical training (McCormick, 1979, pp.17-8). Thus, there can be a tension between the perspectives of doctors and nurses where one is pursued at the expense of the other.

> 'There was one particular case where the night staff were very upset about the management of a patient, who they thought was crying out to be given something to drink, and he [the Consultant] wrote an open letter and left it on the ward for all to see, to say that they [the nurses] were trying to kill the patient by giving the patient fluid. And it ended up with a formal complaint, and a meeting at midnight with the night nursing officer months later, called by the unit general manager to resolve this conflict.' *Senior Registrar*

Similarly, there are many examples of the tensions involved when a doctor tries to continue active treatment of a terminally ill patient which, according to nursing staff, may be causing the patient unnecessary pain and discomfort.

## Training contrasts

Other contrasts between nurses and doctors are to be found in their training. It is accepted that once qualified, further training is a natural development of the junior doctor's career.

Indeed the junior doctor cannot proceed without further training. Junior doctors are required to study throughout their years in the 'training' grades, taking their 'membership' exams and undertaking the research that leads to fellowships. It is yet another burden under which the junior doctor has to labour. For the nurse, further training is not automatically undertaken. It is not easy for nurses to be seconded onto training programmes (Mackay, 1989, pp.77–82), since not only is there a shortage of places but their employing Health Authority may also be neither able nor willing to spare a nurse for a training course, especially if it is lengthy. However, nurses do enjoy the luxury of attending courses elsewhere. They are not expected to do a full day's work and undertake their studies simultaneously. For the nurse, further training has to be undertaken with the acceptance that there is no necessary or automatic financial reward for increased qualifications. One of the major criticisms of the nurse grading exercise which took place in 1990/91 was that nurses were being graded according to the work they were called upon to do, rather than the skills they had acquired.

> 'When the gradings came out I was a resident, and there was a noticeable change. The nursing staff were very angry with what was happening, and therefore, didn't . . . perhaps, they had been taking certain responsibilities, and then withdrew them and . . . stupid little things that they used [to do]. Things changed. They were unwilling to take responsibility if they weren't being graded properly. . . .' *Senior House Officer*

Thus, a Health Authority can be paying a nurse according to the level of responsibility in the job and disregard, for example, any specialist training the nurse has received that is not specifically related to her present post, even although it may be useful in that job and used unofficially.

### Career progress

For the junior doctor there are fairly well-defined career paths, both inside and outside the hospital. Yet nurses' careers are much more haphazard. There are few structured opportunities for Sisters to gain wider experience (Owens and Glennerster, 1990, p.157) and obtaining promotion in their chosen specialty is often very difficult. While some nurses do not wish their employment to become 'a career' (Francis *et al.*, 1992; Hakim, 1991), many find the health service an unresponsive employer in adjusting to the demands of females who wish to pursue a nursing career (Mackay, 1989, Chapter 5). Within the NHS, nurses have been viewed as an easily replaceable workforce (Mackay, 1989, p.92). The lack of flexibility in the employment of nurses in hospitals is to be found in an unwillingness to make temporary appointments. For example, Owens and Glennerster (1990, p.141) note that in one Health Authority, no temporary appointments of nursing staff were allowed to be made in the Accident and Emergency Department, despite junior doctors only ever spending six months in the specialty.

While junior doctors tend to be in temporary posts, nurses tend to be in permanent ones. In their early career years, nurses usually stay longer in one post than doctors. Junior doctors must be constantly on the move, gaining experience in one specialty, then another. As students, nurses have done the same, but once qualified they may well settle down in a specialty for quite a while. (Appendix C shows that more nurses than doctors tend to remain in post over a 2–5-year period.) Indeed, a nurse who moves around too much, who 'cannot settle', is distrusted by colleagues. The effect of the different movement patterns means that the pre-registration House Officer and the Senior House Officer will be the itinerants, while nurses tend to be the fixtures. This means that nurses may have greater knowledge and experience of the workings of that ward and specialty than their medical colleagues. This results in one of the curiosities of the doctor–nurse relationship: the doctor–nurse game.

## THE DOCTOR–NURSE GAME

### The nurse's role

In this game, nurses tell doctors what to do without *appearing* to do so (Stein, 1967; Stein *et al.*, 1990). By hint and comment as to what other doctors usually do, the nurse guides the new or inexperienced doctor so that the doctor continues to appear to be in charge. It is not simply a case of 'making the doctor look good', but part of the theatrical presentation of health care to convince the patient that all is well and 'not to worry, the doctor knows what he is doing'. Part of this theatre is the understanding that the nurse has not to appear to know more than the doctor, though Kerrison (1990, p.24) found that in some instances the nurses will overtly tell the doctor that they are wrong and that the doctor should leave it to the nurse. For the most part, however, nurses accept that their knowledge or experience must not be displayed, if it is going to reduce a patient's faith in the care and treatment they are receiving. This self-denial can be seen to be fostered through the vocational ethos to which many nurses subscribe. The doctor-nurse game is 'an elaborate social ritual that makes an effective communication between them possible without diluting the differences in their status and authority' (Tellis-Nyak and Tellis-Nyak, 1984, p.1063).

## The doctor's role

Doctors, on the other hand, must ensure that they exude confidence for the patients' benefit. The doctor will give the impression, especially the junior doctor, that they know exactly what they are doing: they are in control of the situation. Under the rhetoric of 'the patient's interests' the nurse may deny and the junior doctor may exaggerate their respective knowledge. This game-playing illustrates the way in which an apparently reasonable aim to allay patients' fears in fact exacerbates the power and the status differential between nurses and doctors.

### THE SIZE OF THE WORKFORCE

Nurses outnumber doctors. There are just under 48 000 doctors and nearly 500 000 nurses and midwives (whole-time equivalents) working in the NHS (Central Statistical Office, 1992, p.62). The numerical imbalance means that there are sound economic reasons for keeping nurses' salaries low in comparison with those of doctors. Gender also affects nurses' salaries. Nurses' pay is low in comparison with other service

occupations which have even lower educational entry requirements such as the police. Delamothe (1988b, p.123) has pointed
out that if nurses' salaries were to follow the same salary path
as police constables it would mean an additional one pence on
income tax. The greater number of nurses means that doctors
can be seen as a relatively scarce commodity and the doctor is
more likely to see that there are 'plenty' of nurses around
while he is on his own. In turn this can make any lack of
assistance on the part of nurses seem wilful. The 'isolation' of
the junior doctor may mean he can be 'ganged up on' by the
numerically superior nurses. The nurses may gossip and
giggle as the doctor approaches the nurses' station, causing
not a little discomfort to the doctor. Of course, when two
doctors enter a ward together the same game can be played.

## PAY

It goes without saying that doctors' pay is considerably better
than that of nurses. The greater length of medical training, the
substantial body of knowledge which doctors have to acquire
and update, together with the overall responsibility they have
for patients are some of the reasons for high level of doctors'
pay. (Of course, it ought not to be overlooked that junior
doctors' overtime pay is exceedingly low, so that doctors
working overtime will be paid **per hour** less than nurses.)
Despite this anomaly, nurses are paid a lot less than doctors,
though in the overall situation, both doctors and nurses can
feel aggrieved with their pay.

### Salary and prestige

'Many doctors pride themselves on their intellectual and
academic abilities and are passionately attached to all their
qualifications' (Allen, 1988, p.37). It is the particularly able
school pupils who are advised to try for a medical career (refer
to Appendix E). The relative scarcity of places for medical
students ensures that it is only the academically bright who
enter medicine. All entrants to medical school, therefore, are
aware of this. Because it is those who are used to being at the
top of the class, who enter medicine, the wish to be at the top

*Different worlds*

seems to continue when they enter medicine. Thus, to enter the medical world and particularly the medical world of the hospital, is to enter a world which is highly competitive. It is not surprising to find doctors making reference to the lower educational qualifications required to enter nursing. This educational 'gap' has been held to hinder the development of mutual respect (Kalisch and Kalisch, 1977, p.53) and doctors frequently mention the variability within the ranks of nurses when compared with doctors.

> 'And the difficulty for doctors is that you can't have an attitude to nurses without knowing the individual nurses and knowing whether this is a pretty bright individual or a pretty thick one, and you get all sorts in nursing.' *Senior House Officer*

> 'You see their [nurses] training has been varied, and psychiatric nursing has varied over the years now, between centres. So that whereas with doctors there is a sort of basic amount of knowledge that's required, and [although] it does vary. . . with nursing it can vary by even greater amounts.' *Senior Registrar*

### Vocational aspects

Thus, medicine is seen as a career which is prestigious and enjoys a correspondingly rewarding salary. Nursing, on the other hand, is seen as a vocation in which self-interest is abjured in favour of patients' interests. The 'good nurse', so it is argued by many nurses, does not go into nursing for the money, but because she wants to care for people (Mackay, 1989, p.151, *passim*). The emphasis on vocation has a number of ramifications. For example, how can someone whose motivation is to care for others, be seen to be pursuing their own interests in trying to achieve increases in pay, and to do so at the expense of their patients? Delamothe (1988b, p.121) points out that it is only nurses who take to heart governments' arguments that if nurses' salaries are to be increased, it must be at the expense of other hospital services. Similarly, the lack of industrial action and political activity in nursing reflect this dilemma for nurses. For example, if nurses were to take any direct action in order to seek improvements in pay, then the patients would suffer. The strength of the ideas of service and vocation can again be seen to vitally influence the position of nurses, this time with regard to pay. The discriminatory treatment of nurses by governments appears to have some link with their gender. Police and firemen in accepting a no-strike agreement have been rewarded with index-linked salaries. No such luxury is enjoyed by nurses, even though they have agreed not to take strike action (Delamothe, 1988a, p.121). With the idea of vocation nurses have adopted a quiescent and submissive stance: they are there to serve others, yet rarely to speak out on their behalf, as will be seen later.

Working for 'the public good' and putting others before oneself has been one of the hallmarks of medicine, as of any profession. The increasing emphasis on scientific quali-fications in order to enter medicine has arguably reduced an emphasis on vocation within medicine. Because doctors are now scientists first and foremost, patients may be treated as specimens, as objects to be explored and investigated. The pursuit of knowledge, scientific knowledge, is less commen-surate with ideals of service. Research has assumed a primacy in hospital medicine which may be curiously antithical to the interests of patients. Heiberg (1987, p.1063) wrote that he had 'visited several hospital attics, where discarded machinery stands around under covers like tombstones over the special interests of the passing professors.' Yet the 'Cinderella' specialties such as the care of the elderly and the mentally handicapped can be starved of funds. Money to purchase a one-off piece of equipment is more easily obtained than money for staff to run that machinery, or money for patient-linked spending such as replacing beds, refurbishing wards, etc. Too often, has hospital medicine come to look like a glorified toybox for the boys rather than a place in which the health care needs of the populace are attended.

### Occupational choice

As salaries are seen to bear some relation to worth in our society, the disparity between nurses and doctors cannot but be seen to reflect a difference in worthiness. Thus, nurses get what they deserve and doctors get what they deserve. The constraints on nurses in seeking greater pay are perhaps acknowledged and played upon by governments. Of course the costs of raising nurses' pay are substantial given the size of the nursing workforce. However, the difference between the salaries of doctors and nurses reflect an inequality which cannot but affect their working relations. In April 1992 a Senior Ward Sister is likely to be earning around £18 750 compared to the maximum pay for Consultants, without a merit award, of just under £49 000 – in fact over two-and-a-half times as much.*

Yet the difference in pay was seldom mentioned in the interviews. It appears to be an accepted fact of life. Due partly, perhaps, to the relative improvement in nurses' pay compared with ten years ago.

Only one person, an overseas doctor, explicitly mentioned money as one of the reasons he chose medicine. However, money must inform some doctors' career decisions. That money is so seldom mentioned may be a reflection of culturally 'acceptable' reasons being given for career choice in an occupation which places emphasis on the public service it provides.

The single most frequently-mentioned reason given by any interviewee for their choice of occupation was that 'they had always wanted to'. Perhaps the children's 'doctors and nurses' games are particularly influential! Within the ranks of nurses a substantial proportion seem to believe that good nurses 'are born, not made' (Mackay, 1989, p.151, *passim*), a belief which is linked with the need to have a vocation. It is surprising, therefore, that nearly a third of the doctors who were asked about occupational choice mentioned the 'always wanted to' reason as did over two-fifths of the nurses. The influence on occupational choice of the need to have a vocation for medicine is one which it would be intriguing to investigate further, because to enter medicine such 'a vocation' needs to be allied with a high level of academic ability. From the proportions of doctors who had previously embarked, or wanted to embark on other careers, it seems there may be

---

\*     There are four grades of Merit Award: A+, value £39 880 (185 awarded in 1990); Grade A, value £29 390 (648 awarded); Grade B, value £16 795 (1511 awarded); Grade C, value £7400 (3454 awarded). The above figures relate only to England and Wales. Approximately 35% of Consultants received a merit award in 1990 in England and Wales (Department of Health, 1990).

distinct types of orientation to medicine, as have been-identified among nurses (Francis *et al.*, 1992).

## WORKING PATTERNS

Differences between nurses and doctors are also to be found in their working days. The career pattern of doctors is such that their busiest years are their earliest years as pre-registration House Officers and Senior House Officers. Junior doctors can be on duty for 72 hours over a weekend, being 'on call' from Friday evening to Monday evening inclusive. As will be discussed in Chapter 5, being 'on call' offers particularly strong tests of junior doctors' powers of physical endurance.

Nurses tend to work an eight-hour shift (although twelve-and-a-half-hour shifts are being adopted in many places). Because nurses are usually in permanent posts this means that shiftworking is a continuing feature of their work. Indeed, there are few clinically-involved nurses who do not have to work shifts. For doctors, a lifetime career of 72-hour rotas would be intolerable, a couple of years is just bearable. Junior doctors at least know that there is an end to the excessive hours they are called upon to do. They also know that their 'seniors' have had to go through the same process.

However, the disparity in shift patterns gives rise to much resentment among many junior doctors towards nurses, especially when they feel they are being called at night for trivial and unimportant matters. Scathing comments were also made about nurses being keen to leave on time and being 'sticklers for time-keeping' (*House Officer*). Doctors felt they had to, and often did, keep on going.

> 'If I have got a patient who needs something doing whether my timing is finishing at 4 o'clock, or 6 o'clock, or 2 o'clock, the thing is that I will finish the work and then go . . . for the nurses, if the time is 4 o'clock, that's the stop time.' *Registrar*

> '. . .I can recall where people have just left wards as a nurse, and 'well oh my shift is over' and gone when you're actually in the middle of doing something, like putting a chest drain in.' *Senior Registrar*

The perceived disparity in effort appears to be used by some doctors to support a belief that while **they** care about and feel a responsibility to their work, nurses do not. Underlying some of the doctors' comments about nurses shifts and their perceived keenness to leave promptly, seems to be a belief that nurses see their work simply as a job. Doctors, on the other hand, feel a greater involvement with their work which is part of a career to which they are giving a lifetime's commitment. It may be, of course, a reflection that nurses, as women, do have different orientations to work. For instance, Hakim (1991) argues that the majority of women do have a less strong commitment to work than men and that women tend to accord greater importance to a homemaker career.

It may be quite reasonable, given the lack of opportunities for nurses to receive the training, promotion and flexibility of employment conditions that they want (Mackay, 1989, p.73 *passim*) to give less commitment to their paid work. The certainty that doctors enjoy – that they will have career, whether inside or outside the hospital – must considerably affect their commitment and orientation to their work.

GENDER

## The medical situation

The traditional division of masculine medicine and feminine nursing is being eroded. The number of female recruits to medicine has been increasing over the last few years to the point where women account for nearly 50% of medical students. Despite this, medicine remains a man's profession because it is dominated by men and by male expectations regarding career patterns (Allen, 1988, pp.336–40). There are few opportunities for women to combine the roles of mother and doctor without marginalising themselves in terms of career prospects. There is a very real sense that women doctors have to fit in with or adopt the male perspectives of medicine (Young, 1981, p.152). If women do not adopt the male career pattern with its emphasis on continuity and competition, they are unlikely to succeed. Although both women and men who enter medicine will have a particular competence in science, additional attributes may not help women to advance. For example, manual dexterity, an attribute normally associated with women, does not help women to enter surgical special-ties. They continue to face tremendous barriers when they seek a senior post in surgery (Lawrence, 1987, p.140).

Other ostensibly 'female' attributes are not wanted in medicine. Those who espouse the values of 'scientific' medicine such as 'rationality' and 'objectivity' are less likely to accord value to nurturing, caring and the 'messiness' of emotional involvement more often associated with women. Emotion has little place in the 'objective' world of medicine. Indeed, a number of doctors made explicit the fear that involvement with patients would 'cloud' their judgement and make more difficult decisions about patient care. There is an additional stress for a doctor, compared with a nurse, who becomes involved with a patient. The doctor has the respons-ibility for decision-making regarding patient care. The decision-making becomes particularly difficult if a doctor has an emotional involvement with a patient and treatment 'failures' become much harder to come to terms with.

'Doctors in the main try not to get too close to their patients, because too many of them over the years probably die, have problems, if you got involved in every one of their problems, as an intensive care doctor you have a very high death rate, or if you are a doctor covering a resuscitation area, you probably couldn't function.' *Senior Registrar*

### The nursing situation

Nursing, in contrast to medicine, is dominated by women. Although men are disproportionately to be found in senior positions in nursing (Gaze, 1987, p.250), nursing is essentially a female occupation. And nursing work is concerned with that most female of activities, caring for others. The perspective of the medical profession, in which the diseased organ of the patient is of primary importance, is challenged by nursing, which asserts the need to take care and attend to the *whole* patient.

The 10% of nurses who are male are often given 'honorary' female status. According to Cockburn (1988, p.37), 'the result of the gendering process is that all behaviour becomes gendered and all interpetations of behaviour likewise.' Ascriptions are made of homosexuality, or that male nurses are different from ordinary males, because they are 'really caring' people. Male nurses, like female doctors, have to subscribe to the dominant ideology within their chosen occupation. Those who act 'out of character' are disliked in both occupations.

## Working relationships

Differences in gender are not that obvious in most of the interactions between doctors and nurses. The difference just seems to be another taken-for-granted aspect of their working relationships (Reilly and DiAngelo, 1990). The unconscious assumption that doctors are male and nurses female must form a part of the working knowledge of differences between the two groups. As Cockburn (1988, p.38) has remarked, 'gender rubs off on the jobs people do.' In general conversation, nurses automatically talk about male doctors and doctors about female nurses.

In the activities on the ward the split is more apparent. Nurses (female) wait, for the (male) doctors to arrive. It is, after all, the doctor who is the initiator of action. It is perhaps easier to let a female wait than a male. It may be easier to be rude to a female nurse than to a male nurse in the middle of the night. There is some evidence from the interviews that this is the case: that male nurses feel a greater equality with doctors than their female colleagues. Male nurses also feel that they are more able, and more likely, than female staff to voice their opinions to medical staff.

## TERRITORY

### Geographical aspects

The territorial position of doctors and nurses within hospitals is quite different. For doctors, the hospital is their territory. For nurses, with a few exceptions, the ward is their territory and, for the more junior nurses in particular, the ward is their working world. Doctors will usually work in one or two wards, and are likely also to be involved in out-patient clinics or operating theatres, or to be called to other wards. In other words, doctors are hospital based. While nurses 'belong' to a ward, doctors belong to 'the firm' of which he or she is a member. This means that nurses are more physically restricted in their working environment, whereas doctors have greater freedom of movement, since their territory is the whole hospital. As Tellis-Nyak and Tellis-Nyak (1984, p.1065) remind us, dominant animals move freely in other's territory. In this restricted sense, nurses are locals and doctors are cosmopolitans (Gouldner, 1957). Doctors are also more likely to be cosmopolitans in a broader sense because all doctors have experience of working in other hospitals and some also have worked overseas (during their years in medical training) whereas far fewer nurses have such wide experience.

> 'If there is a problem patient, once it's been dealt with, they just go off somewhere else. They can escape and nurses aren't allowed to escape. They are actually allowed to escape and why can't they say something other than 'sorry' and walk off with a cup of tea in their hands?' *Sister*

While nurses are confined in spatial terms, doctors have freedom to roam. This freedom ensures that doctors are not under the same degree of scrutiny in their working activities. It also means that nurses may be unaware of doctors' commitments in other locations, such as clinics, theatre and other wards. If there is an assumption that doctors are not working because they aren't on the ward, then the doctor's lack of visibility may mean he is more often 'bothered' by nursing staff.

### Territory and working relationships

The differences in territory affect working relationships in a number of ways. Because qualified nurses move infrequently between wards, they are likely to be less aware of differing and changing working practices elsewhere, than are doctors, who may have patients on a number of wards. In other words, the nurses' relatively restricted territory can mean that they become insulated from events in other specialties and even insular in their attitudes. It is student nurses, for example, who are most likely to mention differences in practices, and poor nursing practice in particular, as they move from specialty to specialty (Mackay, 1989, p.34). Of course, as doctors also become more and more locked into their chosen specialty they are similarly likely to be ignorant of all but the most widely publicised changes in practices in other specialties. And the 'tunnel vision' of one's own specialty, ward and patients, to which Bazell (1981, p.96) refers, becomes a reality. In fact, there is often little contact on a day-to-day basis between Consultants, a fact which was often bemoaned by them.

### Ward relationships

For junior doctors, their relationship with the ward is quite different to that of the Consultant and the nurses. Because they keep moving around, the most junior doctors are unlikely to become as familiar with a ward as their nursing colleagues. The different practices and ways in which wards are organized ensure that for the junior House Officer, each ward is unfamiliar territory.

At the same time, while junior doctors are summoned to **a** ward, nurses are summoning a doctor to **the** ward. There are difficulties for doctors in perceiving the importance of an incident on **the** ward for nursing staff when they may be aware of a number of incidents in different locations. Thus while the doctor may be weighing up the relative importance of the different summonses, the nurse is weighing up the condition of a patient in relation to what is happening on that ward. The competing claims to a junior doctor's attentions may not always be apparent to nursing staff.

> 'Because they've got their ward base, because they forget that if I'm admitting patients, I could be admitting them anywhere . . . and I can have a patient on every ward to see, but they only see me on here . . . and when you walk onto a ward they tend to sort of clutch you and say, can you do this, when you've already got things to do on other wards, but they don't sometimes appreciate that.' *House Officer*

> 'I think sometimes that they [nurses] do tend to forget that

they [doctors] have other patients, they have got other jobs, they have got theatre and clinics and everything else to do. We do tend to be a bit blinkered when we have got our patients which we are responsible for, we are only really bothered about our patients that we have got at the time, and we do keep hassling them when they may be dealing with some emergency.' *Sister*

Similarly, the stress experienced by nursing staff who are in continual contact with a patient may not be appreciated by medical staff. Violent patients or patients who are in pain require immediate attention. Delays in the arrival of a doctor cause considerable strain for nursing staff.

### Patient relationships

The way that doctors and nurses see and relate to patients is affected by the amount of time that doctors and nurses spend on the ward. Nurses are on the ward for most of their shift whereas doctors often have duties to attend to elsewhere. Nurses are with, or at least near, the patients all day, every day (although the extent of that contact can easily be exaggerated). Doctors' contact with patients is often brief, intermittent and unpredictable. Doctors are not in a position to develop the same sort of relationships with patients as are nurses. Nevertheless, the more senior the doctor, the less patient contact he or she will have. It is mostly junior doctors who are likely to be particularly aware of the difficulties faced by a patient. This, of course, is also true for nursing staff. Senior ward nurses have relatively little patient contact compared with their juniors. One knock-on effect of the time spent with patients is that there can often be a close, collaborative working relationship between junior nurses and junior doctors.

'I think there is a bond that stretches between the junior staff and nurse that conspire against the senior medical staff, and the middle grade medical staff, making sure that the medical team runs effectively.' *Senior Registrar*

It may also happen that junior doctors and nurses are more

in agreement regarding decisions as to when to stop 'active treatment' of patients (see Chapter 6).

## *Specialties*

Another consequence of the differing patterns of movement is that qualified nursing staff are likely to have greater experience of a particular specialty than the House Officers. While the types of knowledge used by doctors and nurses differ, there is a considerable overlap. Nursing staff will, at times, know more than doctors. The 'doctor-nurse game' comes into play. Nurses will be able to recognize conditions with which doctors initially are relatively unfamiliar. This means that junior doctors rely heavily on nursing staff when they first arrive on a ward in order to learn the ropes. Yet, even though nurses have greater knowledge, experience and skill, the new junior doctor can perform a task which nurses may not, even though the nurse must first show him how to do it. Although nursing staff can be quite confident about their appraisal of a situation and its solution, they must wait for the doctor with the decision-making power. It is the arrival of the 'action-man', which makes things happen.

> 'I think that I would be very frustrated if I was a nurse, saw things on the ward that I was not able to do unless I was able to get the doctor to come along. . . .' *House Officer*

A further repercussion of these territorial changes is that nursing staff will see medical staff come and go. The medical staff have to fit in to the ward and adapt to the preferred ways of working of nurses and more senior medical staff. Any difficulty experienced on one ward by a junior doctor may be seen as only temporary, while it may be a recurring and potentially permanent problem for nursing staff. Thus, perceptions as to the seriousness of particular areas of difficulty, such as summoning junior doctors, can differ greatly. For the junior doctor, each ward is a transitory experience. Difficult nurses and difficult wards may be remembered for a while but in moving on, the doctor will forget them. Because they are moving on, doctors can be less careful about their behaviour and demeanour. Nurses must live with the consequences of their behaviour.

WHOSE WARD?

## Nurses, Sister, or Consultant?

Because the majority of nurses are confined to one ward or a unit, potentially they are able to assert territorial claim. In reality, territorial claims regarding the ward are often couched in ambiguous terms. One of the popular stereotypes of Consultants is that they refer to 'my ward' and 'my Sister'. So some respondents were asked whose ward (or unit) they felt it to be. The majority felt that the ward was 'Sister's' with just over half of the medical staff feeling this, compared with nearly two-thirds of the nurses (Appendix G).

'I prefer to see it as both. But, I suppose ideally, it is the Sister's ward. But that is a nurses' point of view isn't it? We have got four Consultants and one Sister, so each Consultant has things done different ways.' *Staff Nurse*

'I see it as mine because I run it, but the surgeons probably see it as theirs, some of them . . . no, but when they come in it is their domain for the day type thing. You will hear some of the surgeons saying my staff, my theatre, very much 'what-do-you-want-with-my-nurse' type of things, that's some of the more pompous Consultants.' *Sister*

'Much more friendly [here] . . . Rather than sort of feeling as if you're walking on to someone else's ward, and as if you've got to ask the permission of the Sister. Here it's much more friendly, you feel sort of more equal.' *House Officer*

For the junior doctors also it seems that: 'Sisters keep law and order' (*House Officer*) and 'the nurses tend to run the show' (*Senior House Officer*). Consultants were more circumspect regarding ward 'ownership': 'I knocked on Sister's office door. I regard that as her territory' (*Consultant*) Demarcations within the ranks of Consultants were also mentioned regarding the 'ownership' of wards:

'Well I suppose that they would generally be described as the wards of the senior amongst the Consultants, that's the way it has always been, Mr. So-and-So's wards or whatever. And remember we are the ones who have continuing responsibility in a way that Sister doesn't have, I mean Sister in theory does a thirty-seven-and-a-half-hour week, sometimes it is a good deal more than that, I am very much aware of the fact that they put in a lot more hours than they are strictly meant to put in. But at the end of the day they do have periods when they go off duty and that's it, and I think that it is still regarded as the wards of the senior amongst the Consultants.' *Consultant*

In total, just over one-third of doctors felt that medical staff had a stake in the 'ownership' of the ward, i.e. that it was the Consultant's; the doctor's; both, or their own. Nearly half of the doctors, however, felt that the ward belonged to 'the nurses' or to 'Sister'. In contrast, 86% of nurses felt that the nursing staff had a claim to the ward. Only a small proportion of the nurses said that the ward was the Consultant's and no nurse mentioned that the ward was the doctor's. Thus, it seems that territory is only ascribed to Consultants and to no other rank of doctor by the nurses.

### Territorial claims

These findings must be treated with caution. Quite a number of comments were made which suggest that territorial claims might be stronger than the respondents indicated. Thus, a Sister mentioned that on the phone a Consultant would refer to 'his ward'. Or a Sister could see it as 'her ward', yet later comment that 'the Consultant has a tantrum if I'm not here'. Other respondents indicated that the ward 'ownership' reflected the absence or presence of doctors. So, when the medical profession had little interest or involvement in a ward, then it became the Sister's, by default.

'Some of our wards are predominantly Sister's . . . the continuing care wards are Sister's wards. As you come more down the scale towards more acute medicine I get more involved in the patients' care, so probably you run a spectrum from some wards which are almost entirely Sister's wards in which my presence is largely managerial rather than any value to the more acute wards where I am much more involved with patients' care.' *Consultant*

In teaching hospitals, two other factors affected the claims to territory. Firstly, Consultants seldom have the luxury of having their own ward. Rather a ward would be shared with many other Consultants. As one London Consultant put it, 'I share **my** ward.' Secondly, the elevated status of a Professor meant that a 'professorial unit' was much more clearly 'owned' by the professor – whatever he said, went. At the same time, such a ward was seen by some nursing staff to be research rather than patient orientated, in turn weakening the nurses' territorial claim on it. Nevertheless, every day nurses 'hand over the ward' from one shift of nursing staff to the next. In this implicit acceptance of responsibility, nurses underline their relationship to their ward.

Doctors seem more likely to feel that the whole hospital is their 'stamping ground', whereas nurses seem more likely to confine their territorial claims to a small portion of the hospital. A reflection of the way in which some doctors relate to the hospital can be seen in their way of walking around the hospital. Some junior doctors can be seen, the tails of their unbuttoned white coat flapping, stethoscope prominently dangling from one pocket, as they stride quickly to deal with a situation that demands their, and only their, immediate attention. An attitude is struck of 'only-I-can-deal-with-this'. By no means do all doctors adopt such a pose; some are very modest and unassuming, but the spectre of the striding, white-coated doctor is a reflection of the status sought, and often accorded, to doctors within the hospital by all who unwittingly form part of their audience. The caricatures of the *Doctor-in-the-House* films are still alive and well in the wards and hospital corridors.

Claims to territory are, to some extent, about identifying where one belongs in an organization but they also reflect power and the ability to use that power. It is easy, therefore, to see nurses as simply 'holding the fort' until someone returns to tell them what to do.

'I see the management of the ward in practical terms as being the Sister's, but I think if the Consultant wanted to change things, e.g. to decide that he didn't want visitors on the ward when he was doing his ward round, that's his responsibility. As to where the bed pans are stored, that's the Sister's responsibility.' *Registrar*

'Oh I always tend to sort of see it as Sister's. I know the Consultant will come round, like he has his day when it is his ward round and everything has got to be just so, and that carries a bit of clout. But recently we had a patient whose relative has put in a complaint about the day staff and the letter went to the Sister concerned and a letter went to the Consultant and it was only when you realize the stir up because the Consultant is complaining, that you realize what clout [he has] and then it's the Consultant's ward.' *Staff Nurse*

## POWER

Doctors enjoy a great deal of power in hospitals and in relation to the nursing staff. In day-to-day terms, the amount of nurses' work depends substantially on decisions taken by doctors. It is doctors who decide how many patients are to be admitted, how long they will stay in hospital, what sort of tests patients will undergo, and how often observations are to be carried out by nursing staff. Doctors, therefore, have substantial control over the work that nurses do. Nurses are aware of the power that doctors can, and do, exert but nurses are not without power in their relations with the medical profession.

'In a way, in a ward like this, we can make or break a doctor. We can set a doctor up for a fall if we felt like it, just sort of manoeuvre him around and then suddenly 'bop, pull him back. . .' *Male Staff Nurse, Psychiatry*

'Well I think it's pretty awful to say this, but I suppose it gives me and the other Sister a sense of power if you like, because we are here all the time, we know the way the ward works and everything, so the Houseman will always come to us and ask how is this done, how does the Consultant do this, that and the other, and we can always tell them, because we've been here for so long. . .' *Sister*

Nurses do have other ways in which to exert power over doctors, particularly junior doctors. However, that power is limited and essentially negative. At the same time, the exercise of that power can rebound on nurses. Although nurses help to train and instruct the newly-qualified House Officers, it is not long before doctors are asserting their rightful and superior position over those same nurses. Bowers (1970, p.24) noted that 'It must be very upsetting for a sister, after perhaps 20 or more years in the nursing profession, to be confronted every six months by a new doctor who has none of her experience but who has the power to treat her as an inferior.' Similarly, although nurses can make junior doctors lives miserable by 'going by the book' and *not* using their discretion in calling doctors at night, those junior doctors will move on to become senior doctors whose every word they will expect to be obeyed by nursing staff. Difficulties in working relationships experienced as a junior will influence the behaviour and attitudes of senior doctors. In turn, those senior doctors will be influencing the newest recruits to medicine when they are used as role models.

'You see when you are a junior, Consultants being rude to people and you may think 'Oh well, when I am a consultant, I will be like that'. Which I think is sad, but it's true I am sure. I am sure a lot of it is learnt.' *House Officer*

The same circular process, of course, is to be found regarding nurses' experiences in their dealings with members of the medical profession. No wonder it is difficult to effect change!

### Power – doctors versus nurses

The power relationship between doctors and nurses is not completely one-sided. Some senior nurses **do** wield considerable power in their relations with medical staff. They are the Ward Sisters. When there are problems with a junior member of the medical staff, the Sister can simply go over his head and contact the Consultant. It is, after all, the Consultant and Sister who are most likely to have, and to be facing, a number of years working together. Consequently, the Consultant and Sister have every reason to wish to work together amicably and maintain a closer allegiance to one another than to more transient members of the health care team.

'In terms of power on the ward it was the Consultant and the Sister. He probably had the final say, but certainly not without her being able to have considerable input, and with him knowing that if he didn't really come to a compromise or an agreement with her, then his life would be made extremely difficult, because he had to deal with one Sister, so really the balance of power was between the Consultant and the Sister. . . .' *Senior House Officer*

'One tends to have more loyalty in a way, to one's nursing staff, than one does to the SHOs, so it's slightly difficult in that, but I'm not saying that nursing staff are without fault, but nursing staff are far more difficult to get hold of than junior doctors as it happens, so they have a bit of a hold on you, there.' *Consultant*

However, the position of Sister does not itself confer power. Respect is given only to those Sisters who have the knowledge, experience and assurance to assert themselves in the face of medical power. It is only those Sisters who are confident enough to stand their own ground and challenge the doctor who can exert power for themselves. Such a Sister may, for example, refuse to let any more patients be admitted to 'her ward' or demand a specific standard of behaviour from senior medical staff. The doctor in the final analysis has the power to insist a patient is admitted but life can, and will be, made pretty uncomfortable for any doctor who repeatedly tries to ride roughshod over the more senior ward nurses.

Consideration of power must be a recurring theme in any discussion about nurses and doctors, especially within the world of the hospital. The hospital is, after all, an organization and environment designed by, and for, doctors. The view of health care to which doctors subscribe is the one that dominates within hospital medicine. This can be verified by considering the allocation of resources between specialties within hospitals, the 'pecking order'. Least status is accorded to those specialties in which there is minimal medical input. By extension, least status is given to those specialties in which nurses exercise most autonomy and discretion. Thus within the medical profession the heart and liver transplant teams are the *crème de la crème*, while those working with, say, the elderly and mentally confused will be accorded least status within the ranks of medicine. Those nurses who hold views similar to members of the medical profession, may be revealing an acceptance of medical priorities in the provision of health care in hospitals.

## Power and prestige

In contrast to doctors, nurses carry out work which is less prestigious. Nursing is not interventionist and has none of the mystery of medicine and of the 'cure' which doctors can effect. What nurses do is both visible and mundane. It is work that your mother does. It is women's work: tidying, caring, organising, enabling. It comes naturally to women to do such work. The parallel between the division of labour in the hospital and the home has been made: the doctor as father, the nurse as mother, with the patients as children. This relationship may reduce the militancy of nurses because 'the concept of a sister going on strike is as alien. . . as that of a mother going on strike in the home' (Leeson and Gray, 1978, p.64). And although mother may exercise a great deal of power within the household, it is the father who is seen to be 'the head of the family' and who has the final say in what is to happen and who is to do what. In the same way, it is the doctor who has the power to tell nurses what to do. Differences in power and, in particular, in the power of decision-making, mean that nursing staff, even at senior levels, have to await the arrival of a doctor in order to sanction a particular treatment or course of action. It is the medical profession which enjoys (and carries the burden of) legal responsibility for the diagnosis and treatment of illness. No matter how senior the nurse or how junior the doctor, the rules are quite clear, nurses must await 'doctors orders'. Because nurses are not legally 'covered', they are unable to take the necessary actions.

> 'They are a very capable set on our side anyway, that we're just there to sort of rubber stamp things and do the things that technically they're not allowed to do. Erm.. I'm sure in their hearts a lot of them feel they could make the diagnoses, as well as we do, and they know the drugs as well as we do.'
> *Senior House Officer*

In units such as accident and emergency, coronary care and intensive therapy, nurses are empowered to take the initiative, particularly in emergency situations. If a doctor is present the nurses may take the same action but the doctor will, because of his or her presence, be automatically responsible. In other words, because the medical profession has been given legal responsibility, sanctioned by the state, members of the medical profession must bear the burden that entails. This situation is now changing. Greater emphasis is being placed on the legal obligation of nurses to ensure that instructions given by a doctor are not unsafe.

## The doctor as the focal point

It is easy to see how junior doctors can see themselves as being the centre of everything. The doctor arrives, decisions are taken, the action begins. All are waiting for the doctor's arrival. Nurses, perhaps cross and impatient about any delay in the doctor's arrival, will be critical of any failure to take a speedy decision. The doctor learns to act (and it is an act, in the beginning at least) quickly and decisively. Such behaviour is rewarded by an appreciative nursing staff. The adopted persona of decisiveness becomes convincing, and the doctor rushes on to the wards, makes the necessary decision, and rushes off again, with smaller tasks perhaps left uncommunicated or undone.

The approachable and less decisive doctor can too easily be seen as 'a nice person but not so good technically'. The doctor who spends the time with a patient on one ward, may be late in responding to the summons to another. There are undoubtedly pressures for doctors to behave in an illness-oriented way rather than in a patient-oriented way. Doctors have to be utterly confident if they wish to adopt a patient-centred approach: the pressures of the system to conform are substantial. But if such doctors are less than totally convinced about being patient-oriented, the pressures of the job mean that a medical/disease orientation can easily take over.

While it cannot be denied there are many advantages for the medical profession in having a monopoly on medical intervention, it must not be forgotten that the legal responsibility for patients can be an onerous load. A doctor is never really off duty. They know that their very presence brings the burden of responsibility. When first practising as doctors, the extent to which that burden is felt can be quite apparent to those nearby. Thus, observing the young House Officer hurrying to the ward in response to a 'crash call', the pale face and the dilated pupils make the terror of responsibility quite obvious (even although that junior doctor is not ultimately responsible: that responsibility rests with the Consultant). The terror comes from being placed in a position of responsibility as 'the doctor'.

'I was in coronary care, which was really frightening because you know you used to have time to ponder over ECGs. And you had this notion that you had all this responsibility, but you really didn't, folk would keep their eye on you, but it was frightening.' *Senior House Officer*

'It's horrible. It's very scary and you don't know what you are supposed to be doing and you're given responsibility right from the beginning and the nurses expect you to know everything. They say 'Can you write up this drug chart and that drug chart and have you ever written up a drug chart? You haven't a clue!' *House Officer*

The young doctor learns to accept that responsibility and soon takes it for granted. Accepting that decision-making and the responsibility should not, but often does mean, that the doctor ignores the contribution of others. After all if the doctor is 'carrying the can' he should take the decision. The doctor can easily assume because he has the monopoly regarding decision-making he also has the monopoly of knowledge and expertise. It can be easy to overlook the expertise and experience of others and neglect to listen to those who have more contact with and knowledge of the patients. Such a view may be learned in medical school: 'the perceived power differential between medicine and nursing . . . appears to be the biggest factor in the invisibility and devaluation by many medical students of whatever contributions nurses provide' (Webster, 1985, p.317). It is easy to forget that nurses act as the doctor's 'eyes and ears' in their absence from the ward. Similarly, the extent to which other decisions have already been taken can be overlooked. Decisions, after all, have to be taken at many levels. Nurses have to decide whether and when to call a doctor; the decision to more closely monitor a patient whose condition is worrying you; the decision to ignore the patient who has fallen out of bed so that the patient who has 'arrested' can be attended to.

'I think working nights is certainly more stressful and knowing that you don't have the back-up and deliberating over whether you should ring or you shouldn't and what are they going to say if you do ring, and this type of thing, and just I think working nights in the dark and the sounds are just so more acute.' *Staff Nurse*

The experience of stress is likely to be greater in the absence of the necessary power to take affirmative, rather than simply ameliorative, action.

### THE STATE

In analyses of the workings of professions, an important role is accorded to the extent to which any profession has the support of the state (Freidson, 1970a). The monopoly position of the medical profession, backed by the state, gives the profession considerable power. For example, in order to qualify for 'sickness benefit', to obtain 'invalidity benefits' or a disability pension, a certificate must be signed by a doctor. There is no one else who can give such a certificate. The medical profession's monopoly of knowledge and of skills, underwritten by the state fundamentally affects our lives (Turner, 1987).

Nursing does not enjoy the same privileges as medicine in relation to the state. Nursing is subordinate to medicine in the division of labour in health care. Although qualified nurses can practise only if they are registered with the United Kingdom Central Council, they have no monopoly over their areas of practise. In various circumstances, physiotherapists, doctors, phlebotomists, technicians, etc. can and do undertake duties often performed by nurses. In order to maintain its privileged position in the provision of health care, medicine must assert its dominance over other occupations such as nursing (Freidson, 1970b; Parry and Parry, 1976; Willis, 1983).

Medicine can retain its autonomy and independence by excluding other occupational groups, limiting their activities and ensuring their continued subordination (Larson, 1977).

## Legal and ethical aspects

The subordination of nursing which medicine has sought and enjoys, can be used against doctors, especially junior doctors, by nurses. The legal responsibilities of doctors is an aspect which can be played on by nurses. For example, because the boundaries between nursing tasks and medical tasks are not always clear-cut, doctors are often summoned in order to carry out specific procedures which nurses are not allowed, or are unwilling, to perform. (Of course, nurses also have legal responsibilities. The nurse is legally accountable for the nursing care he or she gives and for ensuring that unsafe instructions from doctors are challenged. The rules for nurses are laid down by the United Kingdom Central Council which gives guidelines as to 'safe practice' and what misdemeanours may result in disciplinary action being taken.)

In addition to the legal constraints and the influence of doctors' decisions on nursing activities, the tasks which nurses can do are constrained by the 'nursing hierarchy'. The limits to what nurses can and cannot do have been circumscribed by senior nurses in an attempt to establish a discrete area of competence. However, this same policy has meant that nurses have been limited both in their activities and the responsibilities they can take. (This topic will be returned to in Chapter 9.)

For the medical profession, however, there is little they cannot attempt to do, within the limits of ethics. Although ethical considerations are becoming increasingly important in relation to the latest advances in medical science, limits on the activities of doctors are few. The constraints under which doctors do work are those which are shared by all within the NHS, those of time and resources. There is a limit to the number of patients that can be seen in out-patient clinics, to the number of patients that can be admitted and treated. Nurses are doubly constrained in that not only do they share the difficulties created by limited resources but members of another occupation also play a substantial role in defining their workload. In comparison with doctors, nurses are highly circumscribed in their working situation.


### DISCIPLINE

Nurses are subjected to much greater discipline in their work than are doctors in two ways. Firstly, nurses have a strong and dominant hierarchy controlling their behaviour and under whose scrutiny they work. Associated with this is the rigorous system of discipline imposed on nurses who have made a mistake of any kind. While the medical profession has a formidable hierarchy, it is not one that takes an interest in the minutiae of a doctor's day-to-day behaviour in the same way as in nursing. Substantial control on the junior doctor is exercised through 'the reference' from the Consultant. Further control will be exercised on the junior doctor by the nursing staff.


### Disparity between nurses and doctors

Misdemeanours, and they will have to be serious, will be reported to the Registrar or Consultant as appropriate. The doctor will be spoken to but the 'telling-off' is the main means of punishment. The disciplinary proceedings facing a doctor who makes a serious mistake are considerably less punitive than those facing nurses. Nurses often face dismissal for a misdemeanour which would ensure the junior doctor a 'telling off' and a less than ecstatic reference. 'Bad' doctors move on while 'bad' nurses are got rid of:

'If a nurse makes a drug error it has got to be reported to the nursing management, and dealt with by that side, and the medical staff just don't seem to bother too much. They get a bit of shouting at and it is forgotten about.' *Charge Nurse*

'Doctors tend to stick together, whereas nurses, if I make a drug error I have to report it to the Nursing Officer who reports to personnel, and then there is a meeting where you are on trial, and then if you are found guilty it is put in your personnel record and you are given a written warning that lasts for six months, that's the way that it works here.' *Staff Nurse*

'It is not easy for a bad nurse to carry on because everything is documented about that person and it follows a nurse, it doesn't seem to with doctors. It really doesn't, because we have had, and we will be no worse than any other place, but we have had very bad doctors, and they go on and they continue to do in other places, and I think that is awful, I think that is absolutely awful.' *Sister*

This disparity in the treatment which nurses and doctors face has far-reaching repercussions. The discipline encouraged in nurse training and practice together with the pressure not to become a 'troublemaker' ensures that many nurses do not speak out, say, against poor nursing practices they may witness. The constant reminder from senior nurses that nursing staff are 'not legally covered' to do many tasks (which are well within their capabilities and which they could do in their own home, such as giving paracetamol) must engender an acceptance of being a passive bystander in health care. These two aspects combine to disable the nurse, to hobble her, so that she becomes unhappy to use her own initiative or to take responsibility for her own actions.

Within nurse training and practice, conformity and self-discipline are stressed. Within medicine, a maverick will survive, perhaps even be applauded; life would be made most uncomfortable for one in nursing.

## Discipline, status and familiarity

With power goes enhanced status for members of the medical profession. One of the constraints on the amount of power which can be exerted by nurses is the status which is accorded to members of the medical profession. Great status has always been accorded to those people who undertake to 'cure' the sick. Magical and special powers are attributed to those who have the power of life and death over us (Darbyshire, 1987). While doctors cure, nurses care. Because what nurses do is what women do, nursing is not a status-endowing behaviour, but a gender-defining one. Patients accord greater status to doctors than to nurses. While patients feel it is alright to confide their fears and worries to nurses those same patients may stay silent even though in pain, when a Consultant asks how they feel.

The greater knowledge which nurses have of patients (and the potential power therein) is not recognised by many doctors. Indeed the failure of doctors to ask or to listen to what nurses have to say is one of nurses' strongest complaints. The dominant position of the medical profession is here used to ignore the aspirations of nurses to be seen as equal partners, or at least team members in health care. Scathing comments about nurses' lack of knowledge, the quality of their training or their intellectual ability all reflect attempts by doctors to minimise the usefulness of any input from nurses. Yet the doctors' wish not to cede any of their autonomy means that they are unable to obtain the additional information about the patient from nurses which could enhance the quality of the doctor's decision-making. Perhaps it is asking a lot of doctors, who pride themselves on their independent and individual judgement, to appear to be uncertain and therefore ask for another's opinion. The very essence of the medical profession's claim to respect and status is that of clinical judgement. If, in making such judgement doctors are seen to be less than independent, then their claims to a superior position will be eroded.

Nurses themselves are part of the problem. They too, just as much as patients, are part of the society that gives elevated status to the medical profession. So many nurses are pleased to defer to doctors. Doctors must 'be given their due' and accorded the respect they deserve.

## Forms of address

Tangible evidence of this deference and status can be seen in the ways in which people commonly address one another. Names can reflect when deference is and is not given and to whom; when the relationship is seen as professional and when it is not; as well as the degree of familiarity tolerated by nurses and doctors. For example, Consultants are very seldom called by their first name, even by nurses they have worked with for years. Sisters might say 'they find it hard to use Consultants first names' or 'they'll show respect to the

Consultant'. While first names are frequently used at a junior doctor/nurse level, at the more senior ranks, the status differentials are more carefully observed.

'It is only recently that all the doctors are called by their christian names. All the House Officers. Sometimes the SHOs depending on how well you know them. The Registrars – sometimes – and the Consultants not!' *Sister*

'They [the Consultants] call me by my first name and the other Sister, erm.. a bit difficult with them actually, I always think of them as by their first name but to their faces, I don't think I could somehow. . . .' *Sister*

'If you work in Casualty, very often everything is on a first name basis. I think the hours and as I say the emergency of the situation it often means that, and also the fact that patients are often distressed or often unconscious so they are unaware of all the niceties of the profession that it just lend itself. So Casualty is often first name – theatre certainly isn't.' *Consultant*

Different practices are to be found in different specialties. In psychiatry, for example, it seems that the laid-back atmosphere affects how people are addressed. Thus, a psychiatric Consultant 'would be offended if I don't use her first name' (*Registrar*). The ego-pricking that children can inflict was evident in paediatric wards, where nurses insist that medical staff are called by their first name so that the children are less intimidated by them.

The style of working favoured by the Ward Sister is also likely to affect the degree of familiarity tolerated on that ward. In some wards, Sister is always Sister, to everyone; no first names are tolerated either by her nursing staff or from any medical staff.

'When I was doing medicine, I worked under a very old-fashioned Sister, she is excellent but nobody would dare call her by her first name and she didn't call you by your first name.' *Senior House Officer*

'[Sister] calls us nurse or whatever. We tend to call each other by our first names. We prefer it, the staff would prefer it, we don't say it to Sister, if Sister is there we tend to say

Nurse So-and-So and be calling them by that. But to each other we just say first names.' *Staff Nurse*

Deference, however, is frequently given to Consultants, so that while the Consultant is always referred to by title, Doctor or Mister, he or she may refer to the senior nursing staff (whose names are known) by the first name.

'Because of my up-bringing I have a problem calling people in higher jobs, like Consultants, I have a problem calling them by their first names. With all doctors I call them Doctor So-and-So. Once in while I will call them by their first names, but I never call the Consultants by their first name. But this is my opinion. I just feel that you need a little bit of respect there. You have got to give them that bit of distance. I don't mind being called by my first name, but I don't always like calling men by their first names.' *Sister*

But there are carefully observed distances: one Sister feels patronized when a doctor from 'several floors away' calls her by her first name and assumes a familiarity that the Sister refutes.

Christian, surnames and titles are all used to communicate different messages. They can be used to chastise: 'If she calls me doctor, an icy point has been proven' (*Registrar*); 'I'll use the House Officers' first names unless they've been a bit uppity' (*Staff Nurse*). Names can be used to maintain appearances so that first names would not be used 'in front of the patients' and 'not in the corridors'. As a doctor goes up the career ladder he or she may feel that at their grade, they 'like to keep a distance' (*Registrar*).

This distance-seeking is part of the preparation for the deference they will receive should they ever reach the heady heights of a Consultant's post. It is a process that is appreciated by nursing staff and they will be circumspect in using a Registrar or Senior Registrar's first name. The Staff Nurses will usually refer to the House Officers or the Senior House Officers by their first name, at least after the first couple of weeks when they are finding their feet in the ward. In some places, student nurses are specifically excluded from such informality. Overseas doctors whose first name is often 'difficult to pronounce' may find this used as a good excuse to confine them to a more formal relationship. This can be used as an effective method of exclusion which could easily be interpreted and experienced as racist.

'A lot of them they would respond if you called them by their first name, but we have a lot of foreign doctors working here and it is a bit difficult to pronounce their first names, so you just leave it.' *Staff Nurse*

House officers, more than any other grade, are likely to call the Sister, Sister. While SHOs and Registrars are likely to call nursing staff and some Sisters by their first name, as the ladder is climbed to the higher reaches of the medical profession, greater formality is observed (Appendix H). And it is a formality that is carefully maintained, with a number of respondents, both nurses and doctors expressing the feeling that familiarity breeds contempt.

Doctors' use of first names to nurses, while they themselves are always referred to by title or surname, reflects their superior and dominant position. It is a position enjoyed by the teacher, the boss, and the parent. It is a status game (Tellis-Nyak and Tellis-Nyak, 1984, p.1063) the rules of which are appreciated by all the parties concerned.

## CLASS

Another disparity seldom mentioned by doctors and nurses regarding their working relationships is that of class. As a topic for discussion it caused some embarrassment to quite a few respondents. Some stated that 'they don't like to see things in class terms'. In response to a direct question only a minority of doctors and nurses felt there was no difference or no great difference, in social class. And although quite a number of those asked about social class felt that 'things were changing', there seemed to be an implicit acceptance of some class difference.

While the entrants to medical school may be drawn from an ever-widening pool of recruits, there are fewer class differences within the ranks of doctors than nurses. As discussed in Chapter 2, nurses are drawn from a broad range of social backgrounds. Nurses, in other words, are a more heterogeneous group than doctors. This is one of the factors which may help explain why doctors maintain a solidarity with their colleagues which nurses find difficult to establish with one another.

In terms of occupational classification, doctors and nurses occupy markedly different positions. Thus, the social class in which they place themselves, and the class to which their occupation ascribes them, points to another difference between nurses and doctors.

The physical facilities offered to doctors and nurses may also differ, especially in the older hospitals. Consultants are likely to have their own dining room, (sometimes even with waitress service), junior doctors will have their own common room, the 'doctors' mess' (which it often is!). Nurses, on the other hand, have to use a canteen shared by all other health care workers. Doctors will have coffee in their rooms, but nurses are usually not allowed to have coffee on their ward. In the teaching hospital, the medical school will be a haven for junior doctors, again removing them from the company of nurses. Parking facilities are, of course, offered to Consultants and some on-call doctors but not to nurses.

## SUMMING UP

The substantial difference in the world and circumstances of nurses and doctors was mentioned at the beginning of this chapter. There is little doubt that these differences strongly influence the experiences of working together. The deference accorded to the medical profession and the acceptance of doctors' power and status centrally inform the way in which nurses relate to doctors. There seem to be few grounds for a shared experience. It is remarkable that they can work so well together. Perhaps it is only because of the deference that nurses give to medicine and those who practise it, that any cooperation exists.

# 4

# Overcoming the hospital

Many hospitals are huge, impersonal institutions. For the patients and their friends and relatives who visit the hospital, it can feel alien, anonymous and frightening. It is easy for the patients to feel they are just another diseased or imperfect body being processed by the system.

The patients are not alone in having to deal with that impersonality and anonymity. The nurses and doctors who work there have to get used to not being recognised when they come through the doors, they are simply one of hundreds, even thousands, who work there. Each nurse and doctor has somewhere to go; they know where they are going. However, the patients have to find out where they have to go and will almost inevitably end up wandering into the wrong place and having to ask passers-by in the corridors for more information. There is a 'system' and a geography that the patients have to understand before they can reach their destination in the hospital. The doctors and nurses who find the hospital impersonal are part of 'the system' that greets patients. Their knowledge of the system is power: they are not overwhelmed or intimidated by the size of the building, the endless corridors, all the unnumbered and 'unauthorized entry' doors. It is patients' bodies which will be poked, prodded, tested and viewed. Nurses and doctors are the pokers, the prodders, the testers and the viewers. The hospital is their world and patients come into their world. Nurses and doctors are, in part, responsible for the way in which the hospital is experienced by the patients. In turn, the extent to which doctors and nurses manage to work together affects patients' experiences. Inter-professional relations are not some esoteric add-on aspects of health care. They should centrally inform the way in which patients are treated and cared for.

## CREATING A GOOD ATMOSPHERE

The intimidation which large anonymous organizations often engender can be forgotten, or at least minimised, if there is some place within the organization which feels welcoming. While interviewing in the various hospitals it was quite clear that the 'atmosphere' in each place varied substantially. Some wards were friendly, some distant; some noisy, some silent. The atmosphere of a ward is immediately felt as you walk through the doors. A 'good' atmosphere feels friendly and gives a sense of warmth. Someone notices you right away and asks if they can help. People seem to know what's going on, where someone is, where you ought to go, what you ought to do. They want to help. The loneliness of the anonymous corridors can be forgotten in the welcome that you receive.

The 'bad' ward is the silent, inward-looking ward. There is no-one around to ask and the patients have no interest in you. The atmosphere is gloomy. There is no welcome. There are no smiles and no acknowledgement. The loneliness of the corridors invades the ward. You even feel less well than you did before. You want to go home. And you are likely to take longer to get better here. You can easily become the grumpy, unappreciative patient, uncomfortable in the hospital and difficult to deal with.

### Leadership qualities

A good atmosphere comes primarily from the senior ward nurse, the Sister or Charge Nurse. If the Sister enjoys her work, likes her patients, supports her staff and gets on with her doctors, the atmosphere is likely to be good. If the Sister is unhappy with her Consultant, finds her staff difficult, the doctors unhelpful, the ward atmosphere will reflect it all. A miserable Sister makes for miserable nurses. A Sister who cannot get on with the medical staff acts as a poor role model for her staff (Field, 1989, pp.124–6). A Sister who has little time for the patients will unwittingly encourage the nurses to spend more time in the office, or at least away from patients. It is the Ward Sister who sets the tone.

'It's the leadership ability of the senior nurses, particularly the Sister, I think Sisters are in a very powerful place, they have a large number of student nurses and junior nurses, and they can either inspire them and train them and teach them, or they can be less than inspiring and the whole ward runs differently, it just doesn't run.' *Senior Registrar*

The 'good' Sister will make her nurses and the junior medical staff feel part of a team. She may be formal but she will not be regimental. She will be confident, but not presumptious. She will be approachable, but not familiar. She will be relaxed, but not careless. The Sister and her Consultant(s) will have learned to accommodate to one another's preferences in working styles, in personality and in time-keeping.

Members of the 'good team' will not be paragons of virtue. They will have fights and scraps about various issues, some of which will recur again and again. They will not always be polite or considerate, but they will be aware of when they are not doing their best. They will not be locked into their own self-contained world of doctoring or nursing. And, they will be aware of the patients' world and the experience of their stay in hospital.

## Disruptive influences

Some of the influences on atmosphere come not from the individual nurses and doctors, but from external factors which can be difficult to alter. There are disruptions, changes, structural and imposed impediments.

### Staff turnover

Disruptions to the smooth functioning of a ward may result from a high turnover of nursing staff, for example. This may be a reflection of a wider discontent with the general conditions of employment and work that exists among nurses (Mackay, 1989, Chapter 5; Waite and Hutt, 1987). High staff turnover can result from a poor working atmosphere in a ward where the staff feel unappreciated, unsupported and unhappy. For doctors, staff turnover is natural, at least at junior level. But junior doctors' moves are not irregular as they are with nurses: doctors *have* to move to another specialty, they have no choice, whereas nurses do.

### Outlying patients

Ward atmosphere will also be affected by the presence of 'outlying patients'. These patients, who ideally should have been in a ward which specializes in their condition, have been found a bed in another specialty. Outliers create particular problems for inter-professional relations, causing additional stress. The doctors and nurses will tend to have less knowledge of one another: of their habits and preferences. Teamwork becomes harder. Nurses tend to look after their 'own' House Officers and to be less helpful to the unfamiliar doctors looking after outlying patients. In turn, these doctors seem to be less likely to introduce themselves to the nurses when they go on the ward and communication regarding patient treatment and care is reduced. Nurses have to be alert to the visits from these doctors so that they can find out what is planned for the outlying patients. The standard of patient care can be affected. In many cases it seems that nurses have to learn from the patients themselves as to what treatment is proposed. Some tasks are performed routinely for patients in each specialty. When patients are placed in a different specialty those tasks may not be performed. Being an outlying patient is not to be recommended: you are in the wrong place and likely to be an 'add-on' rather than a central concern of doctors and nurses.

> 'If they end up on a surgical or a gynaecological ward, naturally the attention being directed towards their own patients, I find that again there isn't the same degree of care, so that tends to lead to a certain amount of, I won't say dissension, but I would say . . . er . . . coldness, invariably, because I would then have to go to the nursing staff and insist upon getting certain things done, so it doesn't create problems, but erm.. I think on the whole relations could be better I expect, depending on the ward.' *Registrar*

'[It] increases the stress levels considerably. Trying to get hold of those doctors and sort things out quickly and moving them back to their wards, so that we can get on with the surgical patients.' *Staff Nurse*

'I think that outliers on the whole tend to be ignored. Not so much by the nurses but I think by the doctors. On the whole they tend to forget to go and see. . . or they don't forget to go and see them but they don't see them as often whereas if they're on the ward, they're always around, so they do tend to get a bit ignored.' *Staff Nurse*

'I would not presume to do things that I would perhaps with my own patients, because I don't know what that particular doctor likes so I would tread more warily I think with them.' *Sister*

### *'Insiders' and 'outsiders'*

The presence of 'insiders' and 'outsiders' is one of the most noticeable features of hospitals. The patients are too often treated as outsiders – temporary visitors whose departure cannot be hastened enough. Some doctors and nurses are also treated as outsiders: they are the locum doctors and the agency nurses. (There is a considerable overlap in the categories of permanent and temporary staff. Delamothe (1988b, p.123) reported that two Health Authorities had conducted surveys which showed that four fifths of nurses had a second job, the majority as agency nurses. There are also 'bank' nurses: nurses employed by the Health Authority, and familiar with the hospital, who will be called in at short notice to cover for absent staff.) Outsiders can be blamed for anything and everything, and they often are. As outsiders, locums and agency nurses can act as scapegoats bearing the brunt of any dissatisfactions which may be difficult to air to permanent staff. They can, therefore, service a useful function in acting as an external focus for anger. However, by the very nature of their casual employment, agency nurses and locums are less bound to the hospital or the ward. They are less familiar with accepted practice and their employment means that a greater amount of time needs to be spent explaining where things are, or how things are usually done. With constantly changing faces, it is difficult to achieve or maintain a spirit of team work.

As outsiders, locums and agency nurses can also behave badly, with less respect for colleagues and less care in their work than the permanent staff. Of course, permanent staff who have been in post too long can also produce a stultifying and changeless atmosphere in which bad practices can thrive (Martin, 1984).

> 'One locum said, you know, about getting blood results, that we hadn't given them to him when in fact I had put them under his nose, three times, to try to get him to look at them. Eventually the patient died – that was nothing to do with it – but he blamed me for the blood results not being there.'
> *Staff Nurse*

> 'Because he is just a locum, he's there for a few weeks and then he's off to the next, he never gets a good relationship with the nurses.' *House Officer*

> 'Because we had quite a few locum Registrars at one point, so there was quite a lot of bickering about what kind of treatment was going to be given. Because the [locum] Registrar didn't really know the patients that well and the SHO and the Housemen did, but of course the Registrar wanted this, that and the other done.' *Staff Nurse*

Locums are often overseas doctors who find particularly difficulty in obtaining permanent posts.*

Without a permanent position they cannot settle into one job, obtain constructive feedback on their practices or build up a relationship with nursing staff. Expectations regarding nurses may be different as well as attitudes towards patients. This is a problem encountered amongst European doctors as well as those trained in Third World countries. Difficulties in working alongside women, both doctors and nurses, may be experienced by those from other cultures. And if these doctors are locums, any such problems may not be addressed. The attitudes of some overseas doctors towards women can be both dismissive and arrogant. It is a problem which cannot easily be mentioned for fear of accusations of racism.

---

* For an appreciation of the situation facing overseas doctors, refer to the Community Relations Commission (1976), and Smith (1980).

Reasonable cultural differences can become oppressive when they negatively affect others.

Disruptions are also caused by the movement of staff necessitated by absenteeism. Absence, like staff turnover, is an indicator that the benefits of working are being outweighed by the costs. It means that other staff have to be moved around, often at very short notice. Like agency nurses and locums, these imported nurses may be unfamiliar with the practices of the particular ward. This creates its own strains on the nursing staff who are moved and those who have to try to get the ward to work as usual. The nurses who are moved don't look after the patients they've got to know, but have to look after patients with whom they are unfamiliar. It is unsatisfactory for the patients and the nurse.

'If you have a really awful night and you haven't got the staff on and you have got an agency or you have got someone from somewhere else who doesn't work on the unit and you have got some of the girls who don't like working in the unit and you can tell they don't like working in the unit. You have a lot to do and you have not got the back-up to do it and at the end of the day the patient is still there and you think "Oh God, we need so and so doing".' *Staff Nurse*

'A lot of the time when you are working with staff you know it's a help, obviously. But often we seem to be getting agency and this sort of thing and that can be added pressure on you when you are having to deal with both really.' *Staff Nurse*

At the same time, because the imported nurses can be an unknown quantity, they are often treated as 'just another pair of hands' in order to get the work done rather than being able to use their particular skills.

### Changes in permanent staff

Change of permanent staff also brings disruption to established teamworking. A new Sister or a new Consultant means that new working relationships have to be established. Individual preferences and practices have to be re-negotiated. New senior appointments bring particular disruption because the seniors can so often set the tone or the style for the junior staff.

Of course, the constant movement of junior medical staff and nursing students can substantially alter the extent to which those working in a ward *can* function as a team. The permanent group may become a core, excluding newcomers and even ensuring that the newcomers move on. The 'core' versus the peripheral staff may be a practice fostered by the frequent movement of student nurses and junior doctors as they proceed through their training. Student nurses certainly find that on some wards they never feel included in the team (Mackay, 1989, p.21).

House Officers may also find it hard to keep moving around, never knowing what welcome awaits them on each ward. They are itinerants, having a 'Cook's Tour' of the hospital.

'You up your roots every six months, totally new set of staff, it's very unsettling. Medicine's an unsettling profession.' *House Officer*

'We only have them for three months at a time. I find that is a problem. I mean you have just started training two and they have got used to you and you have got used to them.' *Senior Registrar*

'If it is somebody who is a problem it is superb to see them moving on.' *Sister*

'In the last hospital I moved wards every six weeks, here I move Consultants every six weeks, each Consultant is based on a different ward, and there's seven wards here to cover.. so we tend to fit in to wards no matter what it's like.' *House Officer*

For the permanent staff, the new junior doctor is an unknown quality to be greeted with caution, even suspicion. Some House Officers are paragons of virtue and following them is not always easy:

'You never hear the end of the previous houseman, the last one "he was so good, he was so good", they say. It's incredible they're pining after me in Eastbourne in my last job, and I come here and they give me the pining after the previous houseman.' *House Officer*

UNIVERSITY OF WOLVERHAMPTON
Harrison Learning Centre

ITEMS ISSUED:

**Customer ID: WPP61227617**

Title: Models for nursing 2
ID: 7621115540
**Due: 07/02/14 23:59**

Title: Models and critical pathways in clinical
nursing : conceptual frameworks for
ID: 7622431772
**Due: 07/02/14 23:59**

Title: Conflicts in care : medicine and nursing
ID: 7620489293
**Due: 07/02/14 23:59**

Total items: 3
Total fines: £2.20
17/01/2014 13:24
Issued: 3
Overdue: 0


Thank you for using Self Service.
Please keep your receipt.

Overdue books are fined at 40p per day for
1 week loans, 10p per day for long loans

'The House Officer we have got just now is also excellent, but he would have shone had he not been following on to the last one. . .' *Sister*

Although this movement of staff may not always be apparent to the short-stay patients, patients will feel the effects when there are failures of communication or collaboration between the staff. New faces, names that haven't yet been remembered, preferences not yet learned, all combine to make working relationships potentially more uneasy.

### Ward design

The atmosphere of a ward is likely to be affected by its physical design. The traditional 'Nightingale' ward with a row of patients down each of its sides will feel quite different to the newer 'bay' wards in which there are four, six or eight beds. In the Nightingale ward a glance down the ward means a quick check can be made on what is happening; who is where and who is doing what. Patients are much more visible, but they have less privacy. Friendships between patients are harder to establish across a large ward so that communication is confined to those on either side. It also means that a House Officer or a Staff Nurse can be more easily seen and located. Thus, if a nurse is sitting on a patient's bed chatting and not 'busy' (Carpenter, 1977, p.166) she can be called to do something else.

In the 'bay' system, patients may find it easier to establish contact with others. Being smaller, the bay is likely to have a 'cosier' feel than the large Nightingale ward. Yet it may also mean that there is less privacy in the quieter and more intimate confines of the bay ward. For nursing staff it is more difficult to observe the activities of colleagues or to find out whether they are on the ward or not. It means that the presence of a doctor or a nurse may go unnoticed.

### *Ward condition*

The age and physical condition of the ward can make a difference to its atmosphere. A bright and colourful new ward may feel much better than an older ward with its high ceilings and great length. However, it does not always follow that newer is better. In this particular old hospital, soon to be closed, there was a friendly and cheerful atmosphere:

> 'We all like it. I mean its a sow's ear, its not a silk purse to work in but we really honestly get on very well together – its wonderful – staff problems are the **least** of my problems.'
> *Sister*

## Ward atmosphere

As mentioned in Chapter 2, different specialties have different 'atmospheres'. Paediatrics may well be a noisy ward, oncology quieter, orthopaedics boisterous and ITU hushed. The speed at which patients move in and out of the ward, the age of the patients, and their prognoses are some of the aspects which ensure that each ward has its own special feel to it, with the Sister playing a significant role in defining that 'feel'.

> 'When we've had three or four Sisters of whom one or two would be good, one or two not quite as good, I can tell when I get out of my car and open the door which Sister is in charge of the ward. The whole atmosphere is different. It's like a family where you can have a mother who somehow keeps a calm grip on the household and another one where the children are frenetic.' *Consultant*

### TEAMWORK

Despite the moans, the groans and the mutterings, the vast majority of nurses and doctors feel that they work 'as a team' with one another, at least most of the time (Appendix I). After all, it is natural to have differences of opinion with other people whether you are working with them or having a drink together: the presence of difficulties or conflict is not pathological.

However, some groups of people seem to work together more successfully than others. The nurses and doctors interviewed were asked 'what factors contributed towards successful team working? and 'how could improvements be made regarding inter-professional relations? A great variety of different recipes for success were given.

## Formal meetings

The importance of sitting down and talking with people, getting to know them as individuals rather than just as professionals is an essential ingredient in team-working, at least according to many of the doctors and nurses interviewed. There are a number of ways in which this can take place. There is the formal meeting held periodically between nurses and doctors to discuss general issues and air any differences of opinion. The most common type of meeting is the ward round and the case conference in which the progress and treatment of patients is discussed. Seldom would any inter-professional issues be discussed during or after ward rounds. In less than one fifth of the wards and units visited were there any meetings at which general issues including doctor-nurse relations might be discussed. These 'unit meetings' may not always be the best forum for discussion. There may be meetings at more senior levels, meetings between Sisters, meetings with nurses only, but there are very few meetings where everyday irritations could be discussed. There are many barriers to having such meetings, the most obvious one being that of time, a reason often given for inactivity.

'Every Monday there is unit meetings, [wards X and Y] will go into the demonstration room and they have all the patients names from both wards, and they just discuss that and if you want to bring anything up you discuss it. But . . . . you are all sitting in rows, you are not facing each other, you are facing this blackboard, and that's about it, and you are all in a hurry trying to get out again you know.' *Staff Nurse*

There are obvious inherent difficulties in holding meetings to discuss inter-personal and inter-professional difficulties. However, the lack of such meetings may be critical when problems are not confronted or addressed (Whitehouse, 1986). If there are no meetings, major changes in working practices will be introduced without any advance warning. Consultation and discussion will not take place. The commitment of colleagues to any changes cannot be obtained. No-one knows what is going on or who is doing what. Resentment and anger build up when there is no communication. Trying to solve any resulting difficulties on a one-to-one basis may mean that it is the individuals who come to be seen as the problem, rather than the changes. Any difficulties become self-perpetuating: problems in communication cannot be addressed because there is a failure to communicate. Antagonisms between individuals and groups become cemented. Meetings may be uncomfortable, but at least give a forum for problems to be discussed so that the problems do not become insuperable.

> 'Since I came it has been very very busy, there's lots of tensions, like the Consultants admitting patients when we just don't have staff. . . . and it gets to the point that a Sister is saying you can't bring a patient, they will say yes. Well to me you should have meetings . . . for just thrashing out things that shouldn't be thrashed out in the middle of the unit, and that doesn't happen.' *Sister*

> 'I think many a time, we've introduced a policy in the department, and not told the nurses about it and I had to tell them only while we were implementing it, for example, on emergency patients.' *Senior House Officer*

### Coffee breaks

Formal meetings are not necessarily the best way to tackle mutual difficulties as they can be 'embarrassing, awkward and stilted' (House Officer) so that junior staff are reluctant to speak up. The informal chat, the meeting over coffee may be more useful in addressing problems. The informal meeting can achieve more because it is 'less artificial' (Consultant) and even although the intention is purely social, a lot of work can be done.

There are many benefits in having coffee together, such as being able to voice opinions and getting to know people personally. Yet there are few places where doctors and nurses do have coffee together. The old practice of having coffee in Sister's room after ward rounds is disappearing. There is no time for such 'luxuries' nowadays, the task on hand is all important. The possible contribution that sharing coffee might have in cementing working relationships is overlooked. There are other obstacles to sharing coffee breaks. Doctors can seldom predict where they are going to be at any given time. There may be nowhere to share coffee breaks. Not all Sisters want their room to be used as a cafe, which only too quickly can become a mess when people leave their cups.

'Oh well nobody has coffee in the wards nowadays. This would be very . . . this would be an anathema to our managerial masters, you are required to leave the premises if you want your coffee and go down to the cafeteria . . .'
*Consultant*

One of the problems is who is to make and 'serve' the coffee. Nurses are very wary these days of putting themselves in a 'handmaiden' role. This apparently small problem can be of 'immense symbolic importance' to women (Pringle, 1988, p.20).

'I mean one of my Consultants likes on a Wednesday when he's done his ward round, to have a cup of coffee, and invariably I send him in here to make his own coffee! [laughs]' *Sister*

'In fact the [female] Registrar sort of pours out the tea at the . . . the case conferences, which is quite nice, because that used to really get on my nerves. . .' *Sister*

The need for informal meeting and talking is acknowledged by many doctors and nurses interviewed. And the lack of somewhere to share coffee breaks was often mentioned. The importance of the informal contact was obviously recognised.

'I'm sad that there isn't the time to sit down and **talk** . . . okay yes, about the patients, but also about yourselves and about how what . . . you're doing at home, how your House is, so that you get to know each other as **people** as well!' *Sister*

'The ability to sit down and have coffee and what have you with the nurses and that is lacking I think [here]. So I think the environment very much dictates my relationship with some of the nursing staff which I work with.' *Senior Registrar*

'I think that another sort of thing that is awful about [this hospital] is that there are no coffee rooms on wards here, it is so stupid, everywhere else they all have coffee rooms on the wards so people instead of disappearing for their breaks to the canteen, and the junior doctors stop on the ward as such, it doesn't happen. Whereas in other hospitals they sit down, you have coffee together, and you talk about a night out or something, or a patient or such, and really do get to know people a lot better, and there is less reason to leave the ward as well because then you actually can go and sit down here, rather than go off to the[medical school bar] or your own room or something. . .' *Registrar*

'The doctors usually have it their room, but nurses aren't allowed to stay on the ward. So we couldn't have it here even if we were invited, not supposed to anyway.' *Staff Nurse*

The rules which exist in some places that nurses are not allowed to have coffee on the ward may give a more 'professional' air to a ward. It is, however, debateable whether insisting that nurses go to a canteen for their coffee – where they are unlikely to sit and talk to doctors – is helpful in fostering more relaxed working relationships. Of course, in many places, the more senior doctors will have their own room, junior doctors a common room, in which they can have coffee but in which nurses are never to be found. Common rooms for both nurses and doctors are few and far between. (Intensive therapy units often have shared rooms, a factor which appears to contribute to the reported better relationships in this specialty.) Yet even where there is a coffee room, nurses and doctors may still not mix.

Doctors say that the nurses don't make them welcome; while nurses say the doctors wish to have their coffee separately. . . .

'There is a common room here, they have a canteen which is . . . generally when they go there people more or less segregate into doctors at one table, nurses at another. I mean I don't see it as my responsibility or anything to chat to a nurse, I'll chat to her if I feel like it, and I won't bother my arse if I don't.' *Registrar*

'We used to, when I was here before we all used to go and have coffee after ward rounds and things, but not very much now. The Registrar comes in the staff room because he smokes, so he sits with a fag in there, and the housemen will do, but on the whole they stay apart.' *Sister*

If there are shared facilities, they can soon become a mess and pose a different set of problems: who is to tidy up, who is to make the coffee, who is to organize getting the milk every day and so on. It is a perfect role for a nurse to fall into. Not only are nurses on the ward all the time while doctors are not, but it can easily be seen as part and parcel of the nurse's duties to tidy (see Chapter 5). However, quite a few doctors and nurses do share coffee breaks, if not every day, at least occasionally and when the opportunity arose. The contact was valued and seemed to add something to their working relationships:

'The doctor we've got at the moment, I think she delights in having coffee with us, she's one of the better ones we've got, but they've also, they've got a place where they go and sit by themselves, if they want to be by themselves. . .' *Staff Nurse*

'We have coffee downstairs in the coffee room and the dining room and the doctors sometimes will come and sit with us for our meals or we'll sit with them, or they'll have a coffee. If the boys are on late at night and we're having an unofficial cup of coffee they'll have it where we have it.' *Sister*

## TALKING

It is all very well suggesting that coffee breaks ought to be shared and that doctors and nurses ought to get together more often. But it seems it is not always easy to talk with colleagues. Many said they found it easy to talk to some of their colleagues, but for others there were particular obstacles. The topics of conversation seemed to be restricted, with a tendency to talk only about work-related matters. It was obvious that conversations were often stilted and considerations of rank were obviously ever-present.

'It is mainly discussing the next case or what happened

during the last case while you are having your coffee, you know. There's not much, not many other topics outside work.' *Staff Nurse*

'We talk about all sorts of things to be quite honest. I think some of the staff . . . some of the nursing staff – I get on with so easily; it's such an easy relationship that you can talk about anything.' *House Officer*

'Some doctors don't bother to speak to enrolled nurses, you notice that. They will speak to the Sister or the Staff Nurse in charge, but they don't bother with the opinion of the enrolled nurses.' *Sister*

'I think Senior Registrar upwards, you know, it is more strained. But the junior doctors are fine.' *Staff Nurse*

Doctors' and nurses' attitudes to one another affected the extent to which they found it easy to talk or indeed, whether they wanted to talk to each other at all. Quite a number of comments from the doctors in particular indicated that they had no great interest in talking with nurses about topics other than work. Some doctors would refuse to discuss personal matters, while others felt that they had to 'talk down' to nurses. The comments ranged from the belief that nurses wouldn't understand the medical terms a doctor would wish to use in conversation, to dismissive comments regarding the intellectual abilities of nurses. But such barriers were not only one-way:

'I wouldn't particularly want to discuss with doctors what I did at the weekend, or what I did socially, or anything. Whereas I would say to some of my colleagues 'oh I did this at the weekend', or that. . . . I suppose that there is still a barrier to the extent that I don't socialize with them, they don't socialize with me, so I don't have to tell them anything about me.' *Sister*

'So I think you do adjust your vocabulary, not necessarily the tone of speech but certainly vocabulary.' *Senior Registrar*

'I think sometimes there's an intellectual barrier . . .' *Senior House Officer*

For a small minority of doctors, including some overseas

doctors, nursing colleagues were sometimes easier to talk to than their medical colleagues.

'Sometimes easier. It depends what you talk about. If you talk about the profession, you would rather talk to a doctor, but if you talk about anything personal, you would rather talk with a nurse. So it's easier.' *Senior House Officer*

For the most part, however, doctors found it easier to talk to other doctors than to talk to nurses. 'Maintaining a distance' seemed to be important to some people – particularly doctors – although both nurses and doctors were clearly aware of differences in status. Nurses obviously felt constrained in seeking conversation with doctors, and were also only too aware of the reluctance of some doctors to speak about non-work matters, or to interact at an individual rather than at professional levels.

'I talk to them about my kids and everything but I won't discuss anything personal. No, I wouldn't . . . because I know sometimes when you're just doing a ward, the nurses listen to everything . . . they talk about everyone and everything. . . .' *Registrar*

'I think it depends on the individual, some doctors don't want to speak to you socially, they will speak to you about the children, but that's it, they don't want to speak to you socially.' *Sister*

'We have got some new Registrars now and they are very nice and they actually treat us very well, but when the Consultant's there, they ignore us. It's sort of "we will all talk and get on well together, except when [the Consultant] is in then you mustn't talk to me because he will think I am being pally with the nurses".' *Staff Nurse*

### 'Them and us'

For many doctors and nurses there was an implicit, and sometimes explicit, 'them and us' view of working relation-ships. The dangers of too great a familiarity with working colleagues was a recurring theme throughout the interviews.

The danger of this was evident in relationships with overseas doctors, many of whom were lonely, living in the hospital residence with few friends. A cultural isolation can result in inappropriate behaviour towards nurses. Thus, some overseas doctors were reported to be too familiar with nurses, taking the flirty relationship beyond the acceptable boundaries. There was an implicit wish among some nurses not to be seen to be 'encouraging' overseas doctors and that the relationship would be misunderstood. The stand-offishness of nurses was interpreted as racist by the overseas doctors, which it sometimes was.

> 'During my work I do not talk to nurses outside looking after patients but I think there are some nurses who feel that people like me from other countries, well they make you feel that you come from an undeveloped or underdeveloped country and that you don't know anything about anything. I mean we were doing heart transplants in Jordan six years ago and they still make teasing, taunting comments about "they'd be lucky to be [getting] a wooden prosthesis let alone debating about this or that prosthesis over here".'
> *Senior House Officer*

Many nurses wanted to avoid any familiarity with overseas doctors (yet not with homegrown doctors), particularly in the DGH in the south-east of England where there was a large proportion of overseas-trained doctors. Barriers of culture and language did mean that overseas doctors were often excluded from any general 'chat' and as a result, their relations with nurses tended to be more formal. Racist views are found among both nurses and doctors, the career prospects bear witness to that (Smith, 1980).

Yet it cannot be denied that some overseas doctors' views about women are remarkably sexist. The combination of the two does not help working relationships:

> 'That Registrar I was talking about earlier, he was Muslim, and they have a very different attitude to women. I mean I find that they definitely do not seem to like women being doctors, and you can tell the differences between the way that they speak to women and the way they speak to men. That really bad Registrar I had, he hated women, they

should have been at home and not working, and the way that he spoke to me was just absolutely diabolical.' *House Officer*

'I think it was a cultural problem of doctors who expected perhaps nurses to be . . . take a subservient role and nurses who expected the junior doctors to do what they were told.' *Consultant*

'Even if they are quite Westernised as such, they still think our [women's] place is in the home, and that probably reflects more on senior nursing staff than the juniors, because if the junior is then helping the doctor and doing what the doctor asks that's fine. But if I have to question anything then I am in the wrong, so it probably might be more me than some more junior staff.' *Sister*

It was doctors who had trained in Muslim countries whose attitudes to women were disliked. Doctors from Europe, the Indian subcontinent, Australia, North America and Africa were generally found to be the same as, if not an improvement on, 'home-grown' doctors in their social relations.

## Talking and working relationships

The lack of ease in talking to nursing or medical colleagues is unfortunate because chatting to someone is a way of overcoming barriers and of altering attitudes. It is also a way in which closer working relationships can be established. Appreciating how a colleague feels or the pressures under which she is working, comes from talking with one another. Moaning about the job to each other can be therapeutic. The ability to communicate informally means that 'gut-feeling' information about patients can be passed on without fear of being ridiculed. A more trusting relationship can be established in which you know the other person is going to do the best they can for you. Chatting to one another is a way of reducing stress and tension, because it can remove a sense of isolation and lack of appreciation.

'I think that if you can talk to a doctor you get on a lot better, and if they realize that you are not, sometimes they think 'oh she is just a nurse', then when they realize that you are not just fitting into the stereotype of just bathing people etc. They are actually coming asking you.' *Staff Nurse*

'You see that maybe they are a wee bit down, a wee bit flustered, you say 'been a bad day? Were you up last night?, you know try to get them to talk about something to get their mind off it you know.' *Staff Nurse*

'I think if you have got a good working relationship you all know what you are about, you all know what you are doing, you all work well together. A light relationship . . . makes a good working atmosphere, doesn't it?' *Staff Nurse*

There is, then, a potential therapeutic value in being able to talk easily with a colleague. Developing 'chatting' skills can mean improved communication with patients and recognition of the possibility of greater cooperation with others. In turn, good working relationships foster good patient care. Doctors and nurses who are at ease with one another will be more relaxed, more communicative and less threatened by any suggestions or comments from the other. This must reflect on the quality of relationship with the patient. A grumpy nurse or an unappreciated doctor will find it difficult to switch to being pleasant or helpful to a patient.

There is a circularity: if doctors and nurses can talk easily together, they will see one another more positively and because of that they will talk easily together. The reverse is also true. If nurses and doctors do not talk easily together, their stereotypes and prejudices remain, preventing any ease of conversation and exchange of information and viewpoints.

### Levels of interaction

Although the majority said that some of their nursing or medical colleagues were 'easy to talk to', quite a large number expressed some reservations about the level of interaction. It appears that the conversations doctors and nurses have with one another are slightly stilted, reserved interactions. They don't seem to say what they want to and cannot express their feelings. Nurses and doctors seem to be very uncomfortable with one another.*

---

* Evidence from Australia suggests a similar experience (Kerr, 1986).

The status and power imbalances between doctors and nurses mean that it is often difficult for a doctor to ask for something to be done without it being heard as an order. Nurses have been trained to act quickly and automatically when asked to do something. The seriousness of the work and the accompanying need to respond instantly to requests mean that social niceties have to be foregone. The fact that so many doctors are male and so many nurses are female means that the status and power imbalance is mirrored by a gender imbalance. The cultural expectation that it is men who will tell women what to do goes against the 'professional' aspirations of nurses for equality in their working relationships. The expectation that nurses are there to jump when a doctor says so, acts to inhibit informal conversations or to perceive one another as equals. No wonder they cannot talk easily to each other other, or ask nicely for things to be done, or even treat one another as partners rather than as inferiors or superiors.

These stilted conversations fly in the face of everyday assumptions about the relationships between nurses and doctors, and have provided wonderful fodder for the media. *Mills and Boon* books – swooning nurses and aloof, masterful doctors; *Doctor-in-the-House* films; *St. Elsewhere* – the popular stereotypes of randy medics and nubile nurses in their black stockings and suspender belts. As with all stereotypes they are both wide of the mark and yet a reflection of the behaviour of some. The lack of 'fit' with reality is a continuing **irritation** to those nurses who wish to promote the professional status of nursing. The lack of 'fit' for some doctors, is a source of great **disappointment** that their relationships with nurses are not quite what they were led to expect in medical school!

'[even] when I was a medical student, I've never personally socialized with nurses, hardly at all, and most people that I know, don't either . . . which is contrary to my belief before I entered medical school.' *Senior House Officer*

'I find it quite offensive the popular image of nursing – the *Mills and Boon* literature, I really find that quite offensive, I think it demoralizes nurses and it certainly doesn't do much for a pay campaign.' *Sister*

'It happens, and I'm sure it's a matter of familiarity breeds contempt, I've seen it in action and even some Sisters who ought to know better, they will flutter their eyelids.' *Staff Nurse*

Is there smoke without fire? Is there eye-fluttering and flirting between two groups of people who are often awkward when talking to one another? Flirtatious behaviour could be one of the ways in which the discomforts in their relationship can be overcome. It is certainly used.

### FLIRTING

The great majority of nurses and doctors feel that there is a flirtatious element in their working relationships. However, the media portrayals were strenuously denied. Nurses, in particular, didn't want to be seen as hotly panting after doctors. The flirtiness which takes place is much less torrid: it is a way of 'lightening' the job and helps make for a more easygoing and cooperative atmosphere.

'Absolutely think it is important, that is another way of coping with all the stresses which . . . I flirt in different sorts of ways with nursing and medical staff, because I think it is important. You have to . . . it is a way to get the most out of people very often.' *Senior Registrar*

'I do flirt with nurses! And they flirt with me! I don't mind, I think it is very nice as long as that's it. . . . I don't think you should call it sexual harrassment at work – it's not. It's a fact of life. You do that whether you go out socially or whatever and sometimes it works well. . . . it is another facet of life that makes for a better relationship generally.' *Senior Registrar*

'You will get flirting in any job in any society, but I don't think that it is any more so in medicine or nursing, no I think it is just that if you work with the same team of people you get close to them, especially in a tension situation. And you become closer to that person because you have worked with them under pressure, and I think there is a lot of respect and fondness between people who work closely under pressure like that.' *Sister*

## Flirting has its uses . . .

The usefulness of flirting was pointed out on numerous occasions. It is a way of getting things done, without being ordered or having to order. It is a method by which you can get your 'own way', and overcome resistance to your ideas or suggestions.

'I think the flirty thing. . . . oh, we all use it, I mean, I hate to admit it, but I **do**, (laugh) I mean if its going to get the job done quicker! I try not to – demeaning but I just have to resort to it sometimes, and it is quicker!' *Sister*

'I think that the better-looking male doctors seem to have less trouble with getting nurses to do what they want, than the less good-looking male doctors.' *Registrar*

What constitutes flirty behaviour is very difficult to define. Whether it is demeaning, natural or sexual harrassment depends on where you stand. In some instances it is overtly sexual behaviour in which one or both participants indicate their availability. Some feel that flirty behaviour is sexual harassment, such as unwanted physical contact or suggestive comments, while others deny such connotations.

Flirting means that one's gender is used as a status, rather than one's position or competencies in the job. The hidden message is 'forget who I am, forget my qualifications, forget my power or lack of it, could you do this for me because I am male or female?' With flirting, the primacy of gender status is reinforced. It is a way of temporarily discounting differences in occupational status and power. In a working relationship between unequal partners, it is a way of asserting a common bond. It is a natural activity done consciously and unconsciously by many.

The naturalness of flirty behaviour and the beneficial role it played was repeated again and again. Lighter working relationships work well. It is the starchy and the formal wards where working relationships are more likely to be found wanting:

'When there's laughter on the psychiatric wards, that's when it works the best, and you can laugh and joke and be honest with each other, it's the ones where . . . like the ward rounds that are very stiff and starched, they're the ones that actually you don't get much done at . . . the ones where you can actually break the ice, are much better.' *Senior Registrar*

The 'jokey' relationship, the give-and-take of banter helps reduce stress, it relieves tension and cements working relations. As Burns (1953, p.657) pointed out, 'the joke is the short cut to consensus'. Burns (1953, p.655) also notes the hostility and enmity which can be disguised by banter.

### . . . but can also be harmful

Some people, however, are not at ease with the flirting that goes on around them and felt that it was only harmful. One particular concern among nurses was that flirting reinforces popular stereotypes of nurses as being 'out to get a doctor' or that nurses were the natural prey of doctors. Nurses are very much affected by these stereotypes which can alter their self-image and affect their behaviour (Kalisch and Kalisch, 1986, p.192). Some doctors too, seem to be affected by the stereotypes of doctor's behaviour, not only with regard to nursing staff but in the way they comport themselves.

'If the House Officer sees it as just part of his working relationship, then that's fine, but if by the nurse flirting with him, she is just reinforcing his idea of what a nurse is like. That a nurse is just there to be had by a doctor or whatever, then that's a bad thing. But it doesn't really affect working. It might affect his attitude.' *Staff Nurse*

### Nurse–doctor and doctor–doctor relationships

There seemed little doubt in some people's minds that quite a number of young women entered nursing in order to marry a doctor.

'Some people go into nursing because they want to marry a doctor. And doctors think that nurses, because they are very good at caring and nurturing, they think they're going to make good wives. . . .' *Sister*

'Colleagues of mine and so on . . . who have been amazed at . . . who would not otherwise be considered attractive or

desirable or whatever, who suddenly are invested with this quality of being . . . some sort of prize . . . just because they are in a position of I suppose professionalism and so on . . .'
*Senior House Officer*

In turn, the competition between female doctors and nurses for the young male doctors was mentioned on many occasions. Women doctors tended to be excluded from the friendly banter and the flirting which went on between the male doctors and female nurses. Allen (1988, p.93) also found a hostility to female doctors from nursing staff. A similar antipathy towards female bosses is found among secretaries (Pringle, 1988, p.57).

'I think there's an awful lot of animosity towards a good-looking young doctor – female doctor. Partly because of the professional status and partly because they're in a great minority in some hospitals. They get a lot of male attention from the doctors which sometimes doesn't go down awfully well. There's a bit of jealousy almost, which is quite odd.'
*House Officer*

'Not here . . . I have at [X hospital] where there were a lot of public school, well-to-do girls who go into nursing, from very wealthy families, who wanted to do medicine secretly but didn't get the marks to ever make it, and whose mummy and daddy had always said, well you could be a doctor you know. They don't like you . . . and they also see you as competition for the medical students . . . which all gets very nasty. But it tends to be when you're younger. . . it tends to be when you are more junior.' *Female Senior House Officer*

'Oh sure, not at all, we've been through college with them . . . they've been college mates . . . oh no, there's none of that stuff at all.' *Female Registrar*

The 'special relationship' which women doctors felt they had with their male colleagues is certainly borne out by the findings that large proportions of married female doctors are married to doctors (Allen, 1988, p.19).

'I am certainly quite exempt from it. As are all female doctors. . . I mean it's quite unlikely that . . . quite unusual for a doctor to go out with a nurse . . . for a female doctor to go out with a male nurse . . . I mean, saying that, even one of my housemen has just got engaged to a male nurse, but that is quite unusual.' *Female Registrar*

### Male nurses and flirting

Despite the above example, most of the male nurses we spoke to felt that they were excluded from the flirty behaviour. As one male nurse in the London teaching hospital put it: 'male nurses have a stigma and our status is very low' (*Staff Nurse*). Male nurses were often said to be gay, particularly in London. I do not know whether there is a preponderance of gay male nurses in the teaching hospital we visited, or if there was greater freedom to openly acknowledge sexual orientation in the metropolis.

### Women doctors and flirting

Although women doctors said that they were not flirted with, one or two male doctors did say they flirted with all female colleagues, nurses or doctors.

Without recourse to flirty behaviour, women doctors sometimes were said to have a less easy relationship with nurses. Flirting can help disguise the presence of power, by denying it, in the apparent equality of a joking relationship. The inability to disguise this power through flirtation may be one reason why women doctors can encounter antagonism from nurses.

> 'I think if there is an element of flirtiness, I think that there is a lot of it about, it is easier to sort of get over an argument if you just say 'look I am sorry'. Whereas on the female/ female side I felt there more grudge was beared to be truthful.' *House Officer*

The potentially competitive element in the female doctor-female nurse relationship was only occasionally mentioned by women doctors. However, whether due to sour grapes or realism, some women doctors did mention the double-standards with which some junior doctors related to nurses:

> 'No it's never really bothered me to be quite honest really

. . . I mean . . . as far as I . . . I just take it as 'my goodness these girls are so silly, because there's no way that, you know, so and so that they're going out with at the moment, is going to ever marry them', I mean I know that House Officer quite well, and I know that that's not what he's going to do. . . I feel quite sorry for them in a way.' *Female Senior House Officer*

'To hear them talking about them in the bar belies you know their . . . that they go out to the pub with them and they go out with them afterwards.' *Female House Officer*

However, despite the absence of flirting, women doctors were often said to find it easier to get on with female nurses than male doctors. Here, the shared gender formed a basis for a different kind of relationship not available with male doctors.

'I think that they [women doctors] chat more easily about their home life, I think that they find it easier to identify with each other to a certain extent.' *Male Senior Registrar*

'Perhaps they are a bit more friendly with me because they don't feel so intimidated, I don't know! Some of the men can be quite sort of intimidating and lord-of-the-manor sort of thing. I think a lot of it depends on your personality though, whichever you are.' *Female Senior House Officer*

Other women doctors found little common ground with nurses and were more likely to be disdainful of nurses' relationships or behaviour towards male doctors. The scepticism expressed by young women doctors regarding the motives of young male doctors towards nurses received some support from within the ranks of young male doctors:

'Some nurses, and particular the junior nurses – the student nurses – look up a little bit to the doctors and there's a bit of hero worship almost; however misplaced that is, and I suppose, from the doctor's point of view, if they're young and pretty, they're interesting; they're vivacious, and it's the excitement from that point of view . . . (but) however chauvinistic it may sound . . . I think doctors tend to view other doctors on their own level and some doctors feel that nursing staff are almost intellectually slightly lower down. It sounds an awful thing to say, but I think some of the student nurses play that role quite well.' *Male House Officer*

The patronising view that some young doctors had of junior nurses was appreciated by some nurses who did not approve of the nurses who 'fraternised' with doctors. The amount of social contact and flirtatiousness between nurses and doctors varied with specialty. In psychiatry, for example, flirtatious behaviour is rare, whereas in operating theatres, friendly banter is the norm (the 'stylised' behaviour in the operating theatre has been described well by Wilson, 1954).

'I mean you can be nice and have a joke and that without flirting, but when they make it blatantly obvious, and all the little innuendoes, I think the majority are offended by it, well not offended, they're irritated by it.' *Staff Nurse*

'Everybody is a human being, but I think the *Doctor in the House* sort of thing is a load of nonsense and does grave injustice to both parties concerned. Everybody has fun and everybody likes the company of the other sex!' *Female Consultant*

## Changing relationships

Nurses and doctors have always flirted – if the numbers of doctors and nurses who have married one another is anything to go by. While some are scathing about the attentions which young nurses pay to junior doctors, it seems that some nurses still dream of marrying their doctor. However, the relationship between nurses and doctors was felt to be changing:

'The previous generation to myself there were an awful lot of marriages among the young doctors which were primarily male, married a lot of nurses, there's not that many now, not so many in my group which was about 200 of us at Glasgow University. The ones that have married have married doctors, teachers, other sort of . . . it is interesting how it has changed a wee bit.' *Senior Registrar*

'The thing that has changed more than anything else is the increase of female medical students. It is not long since there was 90% male and now its nearly half female. It is impossible to define relationships of 20 years ago without the dominant male and the handmaiden female. It is inescapable sort of anthropological view. I mean you could not fail to spell it out in those days. It was just that doctors were men and nurses were women. That has now changed out of all recognition. The strain on the relationship is that they no longer find it easy . . . The relationship in teaching hospitals between doctors and nurses was just like an arranged marriage.' *Consultant*

Support for the view that relationships are changing comes from the findings that there is relatively little social contact between nurses and doctors other than the occasional 'leaving do' or Christmas outing (Appendix J). One-fifth of the respondents said they had no social contact at all with their colleagues. Somewhat surprisingly, nearly half of the Senior House Officers said they had no social contact with nursing staff. This is the group who, having survived the rigours of the pre-registration house year, might be expected to be more relaxed and at ease with nursing staff as they have a substantial amount of contact with nurses at work. In the London teaching hospital there did seem to be particular wards where there was a vibrant social life. The different social class of nurses in London teaching hospitals has been commented on earlier, and it may well be that the higher the social class of the nurse, the greater the likelihood of there being social contact with doctors.

'In the ward next door to mine, where I was doing my medical health job, . . . there was a lot of young student nurses who had just qualified who were very keen to get on with the young junior staff, they did get on very well with them and er . . . they used to have lots of parties and that sort of thing in the night, a very social sort of atmosphere. . .' *Senior House Officer*

However, there was little evidence of such a social life in any of the four teaching hospitals visited. Indeed, the reluctance of doctors to socialize with nurses was noted by a number of nurses and doctors (particularly at the Scottish teaching hospital where local nurses were recruited rather than an intake from a wider geographical area). The different social class of nurses at these locations, compared with the London teaching hospital, was perhaps one of the influential factors in the lack of contact.

'We have a night out, we invite the doctors, but sometimes the doctors have a night out and they tend to forget to invite the nurses.' *Sister*

'Down in A & E to give you an example, at Christmas I was the only doctor that went to the night out, now there were 40 doctors working in A & E over the course of the year, nobody else went to the Christmas night out. They went to their own night out you know for doctors, but not for nursing staff and doctors, I think that that shows a wee bit of their attitude that has generally been commented on by the nursing staff down here. . .' *Senior House Officer*

## Benefits of social contact

Quite a few doctors and nurses noted the benefits of social contact, with Consultants particularly mentioning this aspect. Yet, it was Consultants who were least likely to be invited or to go to any joint social events.*

A number of doctors and a few nurses said that social contact was better elsewhere: in other wards, in teaching hospitals, in district hospitals. The grass is always greener it seems. There was a feeling that somehow social contact ought to be better than the reality. People wanted to get on with each other. But the tendency appeared to be that nurses went out with nurses, and doctors went out with doctors.

The movement of large numbers of women into medicine has ensured that the natural association and marriage of young doctors and nurses has been weakened. To the extent that 'catching a doctor' was a goal of some nurses, this goal is now much less realisable given the presence of so many female doctors.†

At one level, it is not surprising to find this awkwardness between doctors and nurses. There are, after all, the substan-

---

*   Pringle (1988, p.55) notes that it is in the interests of senior managers to talk in terms of teams and so disguise the actual workings of power.
†   Allen (1988. p.21) reports that 20% of married male doctors interviewed were married to working doctors and 15% were married to working nurses.

tial differences in class, power, status and pay, as noted in Chapter 3. Yet, the lack of ease is surprising because it runs contrary to all the stereotypes of doctor and nurse relationships which enjoy popularity in the media. Nurses and doctors do not find it easy to talk to one another, having coffee together is avoided, there is little interest in sharing 'nights out'. The contact between doctors and nurses is often strained and a little forced. Flirting is a way in which some of these difficulties in interaction can be surmounted. The disparities in the work situation can be glossed over if the gender of the participants assumes primacy. The need for nurses and doctors to work together is very important. That is why these two groups can flirt with one another in order to get the job done, but there is no flirting with domestics or nursing auxiliaries. These other occupational groups are too distant in terms of status from the medical profession to warrant any familiarity, no matter how superficial. Nurses are the intermediaries between doctors and nursing auxiliaries. It is, therefore, with nurses that doctors need to maintain working relationships.

There are essentially two levels on which the flirting takes place. Firstly, as everyday banter and joking which many use in order to get the job done and make the day go more pleasantly. Secondly, there is the natural sexual attractions of young people thrown together in stressful and demanding situations and sharing unsocial hours. It is from this second type of flirting that nurses can get a 'bad name' for themselves.

Although some nurses complained about the flirtiness being unprofessional behaviour, it appeared to cause little unease and only one nurse said that she found it difficult to cope with. As a coping mechanism, flirting seems to be found in all specialties and takes place to a greater or lesser extent among all grades of staff. Flirting seems to have the tacit agreement of the majority of doctors and nurses. It is easy to be sanctimonious about it, but if flirting does lighten the work, and makes things go smoothly, then it is a relatively harmless way of accomplishing that. At the same time, a reasonable level of flirtatious behaviour is likely to reflect on the whole ward atmosphere. A ward in which staff are too keen to maintain dignity, may not be a happy or relaxed ward for patients.

Nevertheless, it is apparent that there are carefully judged

degrees of distance and familiarity in the working relationships between doctors and nurses.*

There is a substantial degree of informality between junior
doctors and junior nurses reflected in the way they address
one another and in their flirting. However, at the more senior
levels, relationships between nurses and doctors are often
more formal. Where contact is formal and also takes places
within a highly defined hierarchical structure, communication
flow is likely to be one-way.†

These formal relationships are more likely than the informal
to reflect the differences in status and power between the two
occupations with nurses of all grades displaying the accepted
deferential behaviour.

Except in those wards where the practice of having coffee
together after ward rounds continues, it seems that the
informal contact is limited and decreasing. The increasing
numbers of women entering medicine may be an influential
factor. The presence of these women will act to remind nurses
of the differences between the two occupations. No longer can
it be seen to be natural that nurses are women and doctors are
men. The disparities in class and status will be much more
apparent when there is no gender difference obscuring reality.
The commonalty of women is blasted aside by the power that
members of one occupational group can exert over another.
Any common bond which women doctors might wish to forge,
or expect to exist, with their nursing colleagues will have to be
strong to disguise the differences in class and status.

Yet a lack of personal, as distinct from professional, contact
is to be lamented. By definition, formal relationships limit
communication. In turn, a lack of communication means
essentially a lack of teamwork. Getting to know colleagues as
individuals and not just as professionals, means that there can
be a greater understanding and acceptance of differing views
and practices. It also means that communication channels –
other than the formal – can be opened, thus potentially
enriching the collaborative efforts and contributions of all in
the health care team. The patients will notice the difference.

---

\* Tellis-Nyak and Tellis-Nyak (1984, p.1063) have called these 'meticulous
 status games that most hierarchically separated partners play.'
† Mills (1983, p.165) showed that Consultants initated 98% of verbal
 communication with senior nurses.

# 5

# Digging in heels

Doctors and nurses experience a substantial amount of conflict and difficulties in their working lives. This is hardly surprising. Conflict and difficulties are natural when working with colleagues from other disciplines on a day-to-day basis. As in any working relationship, 'if they don't have scars, they haven't worked as a team' (Mount and Voyer, cited by Woolley *et al.*, 1989, p.117). Different grades of staff will experience different kinds and levels of conflict, some more, some less, overt. It is a lack of conflict which may be greater cause for concern.

Conflict between nurses and doctors is healthy, yet its presence will often be disguised. The ever-watchful patients must not be witness to disagreements between members of the health care team. Patients must be reassured that they are receiving the best possible care and that there are no doubts as to what is best for the patient. In Goffman's terms (1969), 'the ward is the stage on which doctors and nurses perform for their audience, the patients' (refer also to Maclean, 1974, p.106). (It is no accident that so many doctors become involved in the theatre, it is a natural environment for them. Where would *The Fringe* at the Edinburgh Festival be without the medics?)

### The patient's role

Patients are aware of their role as the audience and as performer: they know what is expected of them. They know to be deferential when the 'great Consultant' visits them and

deigns to chat. They have been prepared for this great visit by
the nursing staff. The scurrying about before the ward round,
the special effort to tidy the ward and look smart, are part of
the signals given to patients. When the Consultant comes, the
Sister will raise her eyebrows or nod in approval at the
patient's performance in maintaining the drama. The patient
who tries to call the Consultant back; who tries to ignore the
rules, will be 'shushed' and told by the Sister, 'I'll come back
and talk to you later'. There is to be no denting of the
performance; no possibility that the measured progression of
the Consultant is to be interrupted. The occasional 'common-
touch' of the Consultant will be demonstrated when he lifts
the book on your locker and makes a little comment on it
before moving on to the next performer-cum-audience.

The need for a performance (by which the status of medicine
is always maintained) is real. Patients are vulnerable and
suspicious. They read hidden meanings into innocent comments; they look for doubts where none exist and they count
on certainties where none can be promised. It is easy to upset
patients and cause them to worry. For this reason, the faith of
patients in the treatment and care they are receiving ought to
be protected and even reinforced by nursing and medical staff.
But the role of the patient in maintaining the dramatic
presentation must not be forgotten: without the cooperation of
the patient, anarchy would reign. Few patients yell at the
Consultant; few patients swear at a doctor, yet in their
ordinary life, every sentence may contain an expletive. As
children we learn those doctor–patient games and by the time
we are grown-ups we play them by heart.

### The doctor's and nurse's role

Nurses and doctors need to present to the patient a united and
cooperative working team. This is not always achieved.
Failures are particularly obvious when communication breaks
down and information is not passed on from one to another.
The doctor or the nurse can easily be wrong-footed and say the
wrong thing to the patient. Quite often, the patient acts as the
communication channel between nurse and doctor. However,
a continual effort is made to present a united front through

which the patient is kept calm and protected. The way the performance to the patient has been played is that the doctor has the leading role, the nurse acts as the assistant. The doctor makes the evaluation of the patient's condition and decides on the appropriate course of action. The nurse acts as the eyes and ears of the doctor in his absence. The nurse monitors the patient's response to the doctor's choice of treatment and summons the doctor should there be any cause for concern in the patient's response to that treatment. It is assumed that the doctor knows what he is doing and that the nurse knows what she is doing. The doctor will 'leave the patient in the nurse's competent hands' and the nurse will reassure the patient that the doctor is 'one of the best we've got'. The doctor can question a nurse's actions, even express dismay about those actions in front of a patient. After all, the doctor is in charge and the patient's interests must be paramount. Directing the nurse and ensuring that her care is of the best is a central role for the doctor. The doctor learns early in his training that he must appear confident and he must be decisive. The competent doctor does not seek help from others. A dithering doctor does not encourage confidence. Indeed, doctors (and nurses) may have to feign greater certainty about a particular course of action than is warranted in order to reassure the patient. Self-doubt and self-criticism are not helpful attributes in dealing with fearful patients.

If a nurse were to question a doctor in front of a patient, the doctor's presentation of confidence and competence would be undermined. The nurse must take care that she does not cause any rupture in the faith of the patient in the doctor or the treatment. (Katz, 1969, p.56 *passim* also discusses this aspect.) The nurse must act responsibly, putting the interests of the patient first. Even although the nurse knows what the doctor has said is wrong or misguided, the nurse has to remain silent. The need for this silence or biting of tongue is reiterated throughout nurses' training. It is a golden rule. 'Doctors' mistakes are not to be discussed, least of all with patients.' The common concern of doctor and nurse is for the patient and the need to maintain the patient's trust is paramount. The nurse does have the option, however, of raising matters about which she is concerned when she and the doctor are out of the hearing of patients.

### The nurse's opinion

However, it seems that the rule of silence is taken too far. The nurse maintains a silence in public and in private. In this way, the nurse becomes what Lovell (1981) has referred to as the 'silent but perfect partner'. The doctor does not want to hear opinions from those who are not medically trained and who have only a partial understanding of medicine. For the nurse, the public quiescence may be accompanied by a private passivity. For the doctor, the public confidence may be accompanied by a private arrogance.

If and when a nurse does want to offer her opinion she will have to do so diplomatically. The doctor is not used to being questioned and may react defensively when that happens. The nurse must be circumspect in her comments and the doctor will give the appearance of listening. Whether the nurse says what she actually thinks, or whether the doctor will actually consider her comments, is another matter.

The potential for frustration and anger to build up in the relationship is apparent. The doctor is perhaps being given opinions which are unwanted, the nurse offering information which perhaps her experience tells her is important. In order to maintain a display of calmness and capability in the presence of the patient, some self-control is necessary. Anger and irritation must not be displayed. It is a requirement well understood by nurses and doctors.

When asked if they had ever become angry to a colleague's face, a sizeable minority of doctors and nurses said they would not express their anger or marked displeasure to a colleague (Appendix K). Some nurses would 'never dream of speaking back' (*Staff Nurse*), and some doctors would never let themselves display anger, they would 'always walk out before [they did] that and come back after a few minutes when things have settled down' (*Registrar*).

### Anger

The failure to express anger can be beneficial in maintaining a calm atmosphere, in avoiding overt conflict and in the pursuit of harmonious working relationships. Indeed, a failure to express anger may be a reflection of a good working relationship in which more lighthearted comments can be made, yet the underlying displeasure is conveyed. In such a relationship there is no need to become angry. Colleagues are sensitive and responsive to behavioural cues of others. Such responsiveness is likely to be present in the group of people who work 'as a team'. The ability to foster good inter-personal relationships is an important attribute at inter-professional level.

However, failure to express anger may also be destructive. Maintaining silence when one is angry means that the unspoken frustrations can emerge in a more generalized negative attitude to colleagues and an unwillingness to appreciate their point of view. The failings of one individual can become displaced to encompass the whole group to which they belong. Three broad reasons for not expressing anger tend to be given. Firstly, the reasoning that 'it is not in my nature', and secondly that it would be 'unprofessional' to do so. The third reason for not showing anger is that it would only be counter-productive: the other person would retaliate.

'There is no point getting upset and mad at people, because it just puts everyone up against you.' *House Officer*

'. . . if you get a bit sort of antagonistic towards them you know they will just get back to you, same as any relationship when you are working. . .' *Sister*

'. . .you have to get on with the nursing staff or else . . . they can make your life very difficult.' *House Officer*

The different grades of doctors and nurses have differing amounts of power and a corresponding ability or need to resist the 'retaliations' of nurses and doctors. It appears that the higher the grade of the nurse or doctor the greater the willingness to express anger. For example, nearly 75% of the House Officers said they would **not** show anger towards nurses, compared with just over 10% of Consultants. The situation is similar among nurses. Some 50% of the Staff Nurses said they would not show anger towards doctors, compared with just over 10% of Sisters.

## Anger and grade

The expression of anger will also be affected by the grade of
the person who has caused it. House Officers do not show
their anger to Senior Sisters, and Staff Nurses would not show
their anger to Consultants. (Junior doctors would also not
express anger to their seniors and the same is true for Staff
Nurses in their relationship with Sisters.) Respect is given to
hierarchical position. This means that Consultants, for example, may be kept in ignorance of the views of more junior
staff and of any disagreement with Consultants' decisions. The
status differences within nursing appear to be less than those
in medicine. As a result, Ward Sisters are fairly likely to be
aware of the views of their junior nurses.

Conflict comes in many guises. One person's anger is
another person's muttering. Some people claimed they experienced no conflict, yet when asked about irritations with
members of the other group, gave a long list of complaints. To
overcome this, a variety of different 'conflict orientated'
questions were asked: about recent conflicts or difficulties,
small irritations, expressing anger and what they found to
mutter about one to another (Appendix L).

## THE FOCUS OF DISCONTENT

The most often noted source of overt conflict and anger was
differences of opinion about the treatment of patients (a topic
which will be returned to in Chapter 8). These difficulties
ranged from a failure of doctors to manage patient treatment
adequately to nurses suggesting a different drug to the one
recommended by the doctor. One aspect seen as particularly
trying was the treatment of terminally ill patients. Because this
issue is of central importance to an understanding of inter-
professional relations, it will be discussed separately in
Chapter 6.

Often tasks aren't done when they should be. And when
they aren't done, someone has to be reminded and someone
has to do the reminding. Doctors can end up feeling hassled
and unsupported, while nurses can feel like nags. 'Tasks not
being done' causes conflict, it causes mutterings and it causes
irritation. Another widely felt source of conflict is the

questioning of colleagues' competence. There are doctors who don't know what they're doing and nurses who seem to be unfamiliar with the most basic facts. Conflating these areas of conflict are the perceived attitudes of doctors to nurses, which is even complained about within the ranks of doctors. Being treated with arrogance and disdain incurs particular wrath from nurses. Yet it is difficult to take issue with someone's attitude: attitudes are nebulous and open to misinterpretation. Confrontations about them may lead nowhere and may make matters a great deal worse. Nurses criticised doctors' attitudes towards patients frequently. Again, it isn't easy to complain about the indefinable rudeness or shortness in dealing with a patient. However, anger would be expressed about particular incidents, when, for example, patients are given bad news in a brusque and cursory fashion.

'It often comes down to people thinking that some doctors are very sort of arrogant and don't listen to what they are saying . . . and that's probably the biggest thing, and that can be with all staff, not just the junior house staff or the Senior House Officers, probably most of them [these conflicts] are with the Consultants.' *Senior House Officer*

'Dressings on people's legs and that, the doctor will maybe want to use the old fashioned, the things that they have been used to, some nurses have done research into dressings and things like that and when to use the new techniques, sometimes that can cause conflict between them.' *Staff Nurse*

'When I was in Geriatrics they [nurses] used to think that we, as a team, discharged people home too early, but then it's the bed problem now. In a perfect world that wouldn't exist. But with the constraints that are put upon us, it's not so easy. It all comes down to care I think doesn't it? They don't think we are giving the patient enough care.' *Senior House Officer*

'Here I would say it would be more to do with the patients, and 'you know what Doctor-So-and-so did to Mrs So-and-so, you know she came in and gave her IV drug in her bath', and all these sort of things.' *Staff Nurse*

'Well I think that happens sometimes on both sides, like when they ask for things to be done and they aren't done by the nursing side – they do get cross, especially the junior doctors, they're the ones who sort of get the stick at the end of the day, when things aren't done by nursing staff.' *Staff Nurse*

'I think one of the things you hear a lot is, well two things really: sometimes doctors hide things from the patients so you can't come out and tell them they've got cancer and that they're dying. You can hide it from their relatives sometimes which I think is very wrong or to stand there in the ward and let every other patient hear what they've got to say. "I'm sorry my dear but you've got cancer". I think both those two things are wrong. I think you hear a lot of people "oh Mr. So-and-so said such and such a thing in the middle of the ward the other day".' *Sister*

## CONFLICT IS UNAVOIDABLE

To a great extent, these and many other conflicts, cannot be avoided. There are at least four reasons why such conflict is inevitable and sometimes, quite reasonable. Firstly, there are the constraints in 'the system'. These are the constraints under which the NHS has to function and which affect all those who work in it. The financial constraints and guidelines imposed on the NHS have been accompanied by pressures to give value for money. Doctors have been exhorted to reduce waiting lists and to increase patient throughput. In turn, doctors' attempts to treat more patients has meant that they and nursing staff are working under increased pressure. Although 'lists going over' in operating theatres is not a new complaint, it is now being voiced particularly strongly. The need to reduce waiting lists has meant that surgeons try to squeeze as many patients as they can in to their lists of patients to be operated on. Nurses are frequently being asked to work beyond their finishing time. For the surgeon who has the theatre for one or two days each week, working over is not unreasonable. For nurses who work in that theatre five days a week, the same request every day becomes a source of real conflict.

As mentioned previously, outlying patients are another

constraint within 'the system' causing additional problems of communication and cooperation. Similarly, locum doctors and agency nurses, people who are not part of the usual team, can considerably add to the level of conflict experienced. The 'outsiders' can be used as scapegoats for the frustrations for medical and nursing staff which the pressures generate. The reduced commitment of temporary staff means that attitudes and behaviour are less placatory, sometimes even confrontational. The greater pressure on nursing staff, having to look after increasing numbers of patients for shorter and shorter periods of time means that they are likely to feel overworked and stressed (Mackay, 1989, pp.55–71). Not surprisingly, nurses are increasingly unable to assist junior doctors when they become overloaded. Any perceived slacking by junior doctors such as having a coffee at an inappropriate moment can harden nurses' attitudes to them as a group. The inability to help can soon become an unwillingness to help, even when the pressure recedes. The often-heard complaint that 'things that they had been asked to do hadn't been done', reflects an inability and also an associated reluctance to help.

## INDIVIDUAL PERSONALITIES

In turn, the response to the pressures in part depends on individual personalities as well as a willingness to appreciate the difficulties being faced by colleagues. Difficult people are to be found in every walk of life: the rude, the lazy, the superior and the obnoxious individuals whose attitudes make working together very hard. The presence of difficult and abrasive people is a second reason why conflict is natural and inevitable. However, the argument that conflicts stem from awkward individuals loses some of its credibility when the majority of individuals (doctors or nurses) are seen as difficult or rude. For example, one Senior House Officer said that nurses would mutter about those doctors 'who were rude and unpleasant and did things without due consideration, which is probably about half.' Thus, the excuses of 'personality' have to be rejected and attention re-directed to issues of professional demeanour. Leeson and Gray (1978, pp.47–8) put it well:

'Explanations involving personal attitudes or individual failings are no doubt relevant in some instances, but are on the
whole totally inadequate, defeatist, sexist, and offer no
practical solution at all.'

## Negative attitudes

A third reason why conflict and difficulties are inevitable is
the experience of negative attitudes to nurses, which give rise
to keenly felt antagonisms. The 'superior' demeanour of many
doctors is often carefully groomed at medical school. It is a
way in which the ascendancy of the medical profession can be
asserted on a daily basis. As noted earlier, this superior and
confident demeanour is partly demanded by the patient.
However, in asserting their superiority, doctors are correspondingly distancing themselves from nurses and refuting
the claims of nurses to a professional status. This superior
demeanour is often accompanied by an unwillingness to listen
to nurses' views or to seek information about patients from
them. One response to this from nurses is to question the
decisions of junior doctors. After all, if they are not using all
the available information in reaching their decisions, then
what sort of doctor are they? Doctors greatly resent their
decisions being questioned by nurses. Who, after all, is meant
to be in charge? Whose name is on the prescription chart? The
perception that some nurses are trying to take over the
doctor's role results in an even greater reluctance to obtain a
nursing input into medical decisions. It needs to be emphasized that this questioning takes place only at junior doctor
level. It does not take place in front of the patient and seems to
be of the ego-pricking variety. It is part of the 'retaliations' by
which nurses can make a junior doctor's life very uncomfortable. Junior doctors are particularly vulnerable in their earliest
days. They are seeking to establish themselves as competent
doctors, but if they adopt a superior attitude too early, they
can be punished by the nursing staff. Respect has to be
earned, it is not automatically given. Queries about a doctor's
competence is an easy way to undermine his or her
confidence.

Another response to the attempts by nurses to have their
views listened to, is for the doctors to point to the great

variation of ability among nurses. Thus, one nurse is seen as being highly intelligent and another as 'brain-dead'. The variability in nurses' approach and competency is used to support the argument that it is only particular nurses, whom one respects, whose opinions will be sought. The newly-arrived nurse, whatever her qualifications, will find her views unheard. As will the possible contributions of domestics and nursing auxiliaries who may well have particularly relevant information about a patient (Hart, 1991; Skeet and Elliott, 1978). She has to prove herself, over time, in order to win the ear of the doctor. A frustrating situation for the highly skilled and experienced nurse who has recently moved to a new hospital. It would be too easy for such a nurse to ridicule some medical decisions which fail to take account of nurses' observations regarding the patient.

### Differing views

A fourth reason for the natural existence of conflict is the different views of health care held within nursing and medicine. The need for the medical profession to do all that is possible for each and every patient is laudable. The need for the nursing profession to ensure that patients' emotional and social needs are met is laudable; unfortunately, the two are not always compatible. It is, however, a difference in perspective which can contribute positively to the debates regarding the appropriate care for patients. The presence and (non-public) expression of countering views regarding what is best for a patient means that decisions are taken after careful delibera-tion and the consideration of alternatives. Thus, questions as to whether to treat or not to treat; whether to use one treatment or another; whether the patient is able to look after his or her self at home, can all be addressed from different viewpoints. In turn, while decision-making regarding patient management can become less straightforward, the patient's interests can be more carefully considered.

These four aspects underline the unavoidability of conflict: the constraints of the system, the difficult personalities, the wish to defend one's professional status and the different views of the patient and health care. Differences of power and status themselves do not seem to lead to conflict. It is only when one group visibly tries to dominate the other that conflicts emerge.

## Nurse–Consultant conflict

Very seldom do nurses mention overt conflict with Consultants or Senior Registrars. There are few nurses, and they would tend to be the more senior or nurses who have trained overseas, who would express anger to a Consultant's face. Nurses who have trained in countries like Australia and New Zealand offer a particular challenge to nurses and doctors alike in the UK. (We did not interview any nurses who had trained in the Third World.) It is these overseas-trained nurses who will 'cock-a-snook' at the traditions of deference they encounter here. They will talk back to doctors, they will question doctors' decisions with impunity, and they will offer their opinions with alacrity. These overseas nurses may show none of the deference and quiescence of the British-trained nurse. They are not part of the class and status system. Because of that, these nurses are treated differently, enjoying a more equal relationship with the medical profession; and they treat doctors differently, as equals. These nurses can be particularly scathing about homegrown nurses' refusal to question doctors' decisions or to take responsibility. Thus, homegrown nurses can be described as 'doormats' for doctors, playing their 'little nursey bit' (*Staff Nurse*). Doctors will be respected by these overseas nurses but only for their competence, not by dint of their position. At the same time, these overseas nurses would be much more willing to take over medical tasks currently being undertaken by nurses in this country. Needless to say, these overseas nurses experience conflict when they work in UK hospitals, but the conflict tends to be more with other nurses than with members of the medical profession.

Consultants will be muttered about and their differing 'little ways' can cause irritation. But there are extremely few nurses who will become angry to a Consultant's face and not so many who will question anything a Consultant says. But at a junior doctor level the experience of conflict is more likely. Junior doctors have less status and power, as well as greater contact with nurses. Consultants are permanent and that means that both they and nursing staff have to learn to live with one another. Nurses make accommodations which would not be contemplated for more junior doctors. Consultants themselves would be extremely surprised if a junior nurse were to question their practices or to express irritation.

## Doctor–nurse conflict

Junior doctors would think twice about expressing anger to a Senior Sister who has, after all, seen many junior doctors come and go. She is likely to have an established and viable working relationship with the Consultant(s) of which junior doctors are only too aware. Senior Sisters are likely to have withering ways with junior doctors who are too cocky or insolent. Similarly, it may be difficult to express irritation to Sisters, given the potential for misunderstanding or retaliation which such expression might evoke. It is junior nurses and junior doctors who are most likely to express and to be the recipients of frustration, anger and conflict.

## 'On call'

There are three particularly interesting areas in which conflict is experienced at junior doctor and nurse level. Firstly, the system of junior doctors being on call. Having 'a bleep' and being called was a never-ending source of dissatisfaction from junior doctors. Junior doctors complain along the lines of: 'Nurses bleep us for the most trivial things. Its absolutely pathetic when they phone us about giving two paracetamol. They never seem to use their initiative or be willing to take responsibility themselves. Nurses are so unhelpful and don't appreciate how hard we work or the hours that we put in. If nurses did appreciate it, then they wouldn't bleep us so often. And then we wouldn't be so bad-tempered all the time.'

There is an acceptance among senior doctors that they will always work on an on-call basis. It is an aspect of their job never mentioned by Consultants, yet it is one which would strike most of us as extremely onerous. The possibility of being called is an always present threat to any activity: the intrusiveness of which is only fully appreciated by those who have experienced it. The special aura which doctors enjoy may be a reflection of the always-present expectation that they will be called upon. When the question is asked: 'is there a doctor in the house?', there must be a special *frisson* in being the one who can respond to the emergency.

On the other hand, nurses complain that doctors are slow to respond to their bleeps and don't come when they are called. 'They are never there when you want them and when you do phone them up, doctors are abusive and rude. Doctors don't seem to realize that we phone them when we are worried and that if we weren't worried we wouldn't have phoned them. There's no need for them to treat us as though we were idiots. No wonder some nurses phone them up for small things.' These are caricatures of the views of nurses and doctors regarding the bleep and doctors being on call, but they give a composite picture of their experiences (Appendix M). Women doctors were more likely to complain about being called or bleeped than their male colleagues.

> 'The strain of being on call all weekends, and being up all hours, and then they are still expected to be smiling in the morning when you come in all fresh, and you think 'old grumpy', you know, but they have had a hard time.' *Staff Nurse*

> 'We are at the mercy of our pagers. Which, instead of being used as they were initially conceived of as a way of contacting doctors in an emergency, they are used for every single pathetic little problem that is at hand. That is a major bone of contention.' *House Officer*

> 'They almost line up beside a phone and call you one by one – at least that's what it feels like, instead of one person co-ordinating relationships with the doctors and deciding what needs to be done and getting somebody to make one call.' *House Officer*

> 'But if you are down having your dinner, or even in your bed and they phone and say someone's not very well, the least I expect is for them to do the basic nursing observations which is just pulse, blood pressure tempera-ture, respiratory rate. So that gets me quite annoyed. . .' *House Officer*

> 'You just want to crawl away under a stone you know when

you hear some [calls] they've got, but they do get bleeped you know for the silliest of things.' *Sister*

'When I get frustrated and angry, is when the new night shift comes on, and they're bright as buttons, and I've been on for the whole week-end and it's Sunday afternoon, and it's the late shift, and I've been doing obstetrics, and I've been up all night, and they're breezy as hell, and they get stroppy then if I seem to be less charming, less something not quite as, you know, your usual self, or whatever, and there isn't an appreciation.' *Senior House Officer*

'I think it is a lot to do with the fact that they're . . . the majority of the people that are looking after . . . the patients, are so young! The student nurses can be eighteen, nineteen . . . and they're looking after sick people and they don't necessarily stop and think about using their common sense. I think it's surprising how many of them **do** actually.' *Sister*

'One can understand the stress that they get, then, because they can't do anything, they can't have their lunch, they can't go to the lavatory even, because the bleep goes off all the time . . . and when it's stupid questions in the middle of the night, you can understand why they get ratty.' *Sister*

An aspect which compounds the miseries of being on call is that nurses are meant to inform doctors when, for example, a patient's test results return from the laboratory. Even although the results may be 'normal', the nurse ought to tell the doctor. The nurse, going through her paperwork in the middle of the night, may find test results about which the doctor has not been told. In phoning them in the middle of the night, the nurse is following the letter, but not the spirit, of the rule that the doctor must be informed. It is a way in which nurses can absolve themselves from responsibility. Once 'doctor informed' is written in the patient's notes, the matter is no longer the responsibility of the nurse. The doctor, woken to be told that some test results are normal, is quite reasonably going to be furious and the nurse perhaps deserves what she gets. However, such a phone call may be the nurse getting her own back on a doctor who cannot treat her with any civility or courtesy. It is at night that the junior doctor is at his most vulnerable and nurses know it.

Because of this vulnerability, guidelines have been given as to when doctors are to be called at night. In many hospitals there are rules as to which grade of nurse is to be allowed to call a doctor during the night. Practices vary considerably. For example, in some units only the night Sister can summon a doctor, while in other units, a Staff Nurse can call a doctor herself.

### Verbal instructions

One way in which the burden of being 'on call' can be reduced for junior doctors is nurses being prepared to take verbal instructions. A nurse may not, even in an emergency situation, administer a drug for which the patient has not previously been prescribed. This practice is deemed unreliable and potentially hazardous to the patient by the United Kingdom Central Council, the body which lays down guidelines as to what nurses can and cannot do. If a doctor is phoned during the night, the nurse will inform him of the condition of the patient and the doctor may then suggest that the nurse increase the dosage of a particular drug. If the nurse agrees to do so, then she has taken a verbal instruction.

She is not really supposed to do this, or at least not on her own. Any change in medication ought to be written up by the doctor before the nurse administers the drug. (Drugs can be written up by a doctor for a patient *pro re nata*, which means that the drugs can be administered as required or whenever necessary. There will be no reason for the doctor to be called if drugs have been so prescribed.) If the change is not written up in the patient's notes and the nurse administers the drugs, then she becomes legally responsible for the action. If the doctor does not write up the drugs administered the nurse will be in serious trouble. If the nurse agrees to take 'a verbal' she must be absolutely certain that the doctor will, in fact, write the drug up in the patient's notes in the morning. In essential circumstances, if the nurse repeats the doctors instructions back to him, over the phone in the presence of another nurse, and then records it there will be an independent witness to her action.

Some nurses refuse to take verbals at all. Others will do so if they trust the doctor and have a good working relationship.

Others take verbals as long as they have a witness to their telephone conversation. There were substantial variations in the experiences among the nurses and doctors interviewed regarding verbals. Predictably, practices varied from ward to ward, specialty to specialty, and nurse to nurse. One of the deciding factors was the extent to which nurses appreciated, and more importantly sympathized, with the workload of a junior doctor. For some junior doctors a 'good nurse' was one who would take a verbal. The need for trust is obvious and trust is something which takes time to establish. The newly-qualified House Officer will have to get up out of bed no matter what. For the House Officer who has been qualified for a few months, if he has managed to develop a rapport with the nursing staff and has decided which nurses' judgement he can trust, his nocturnal visits can be minimized. While some nurses were circumspect about taking 'verbals', so were some junior doctors:

> 'But it's very difficult to practice medicine over the telephone at all . . . the big problem about being called out in the night and generally in medicine is that really it's almost impossible ever to say no or deal with a problem over the telephone unless you have tremendous confidence. . . . even in the person that you're talking to, so you know what they are telling you is right, and you trust what they're telling you so you can say okay, well I'm not worried about that, and just do this. . .' *Senior Registrar*

> '[Here] they're much more lax and they take verbal messages. . .' *Senior House Officer*

> 'You have to go and definitely decide that there isn't a problem. You can't just do that at a distance so you have to physically go and do some work to find out that it is not a problem.' *Senior House Officer*

There is trust necessary in giving and in taking 'verbals'. The doctor has to be able to trust the nurse's report on and evaluation of the patient's condition. The doctor must feel confident in not going to the ward. If he fails to visit the ward, having given a verbal instruction, and something happens to the patient, the junior will be in trouble. A severe 'talking to' is likely to be administered by the doctor's seniors, at each

level. Some senior doctors have particular skills in 'demolish-
ing' a junior doctor, a practice honed over the years during
ward rounds and much feared by the junior doctor. Although
the extent of the discipline exerted on junior doctors is less
severe than that exerted over nurses (see Chapter 9), acute
discomfiture and embarrassment are frequently administered.

### The nursing hierarchy

The frustration of being called in the middle of the night about
trivial things was often blamed on the 'nursing hierarchy'.
Thus, it was the nursing hierarchy, rather than nurses
themselves which was identified as wanting to limit the
responsibility and tasks undertaken by nurses.

'I know that the nursing hierarchy make it impossible for
them, but like giving out non-prescription drugs they still
would have to phone you in the middle of the night, at three
in the morning to say so-and-so has wakened up with a
headache and they are not written up for paracetamol,
which is I think frustrating for them and they have to cover
themselves.' *Senior House Officer*

'The amount of practical things that nurses can do tend to be
so limited. Again, this is the nursing hierarchy. There is no
conceivable reason why nurses shouldn't be giving IV
drugs. And to rouse junior doctors out of bed in the wee
hours of the morning to do that is just inexcusable.'
*Consultant*

'To call these people managers is actually a bad use of the
term manager, somebody who is a manager manages
people, these people don't rule people, they regulate people.'
*Consultant*

It is senior doctors who are most like to blame Nursing
Officers and the 'nursing hierarchy' for nurses' unwillingness
or inability to undertake junior doctors' tasks. At issue is the
power being exerted over nurses, which comes from within
nursing rather than from the medical profession. Senior
doctors particularly resent the lack of control they have over
nurses in this area. To some extent, Nursing Officers are used

as a scapegoat on which to lay the blame for junior doctors' inability to keep up with the increasing demands made upon them. As scapegoats, Nursing Officers may perform a useful function in directing attention away from the nurses on the wards (Chapter 10).

## TIDYING

Another area which causes particular frustrations for nurses is that of tidying. Tidying was not an issue that emerged spontaneously from the interviews. Resentment and irritation at being expected to tidy up after doctors only emerged when the question was specifically asked in the interviews. It wasn't something which was described in response to questions about conflict or anger. This may be because tidying is an accepted part of nurses' work. What isn't accepted, at least by some nurses, is that they should tidy up after doctors. When doctors perform a procedure, like taking a blood sample, they sometimes leave the used needle and all the bits and pieces on the patients' beds. Such untidiness can be dangerous: a nurse or a patient may inadvertently stab themselves with a used needle. There are explicit guidelines about the disposal of 'sharps'. Great care ought to be taken in their disposal. However, some doctors seem to think that nurses are just waiting to pick up everything they leave behind. It's not just used needles which have to be cleared away and tidied, it's other things like patients' notes and coffee cups.

The doctors say that when they are so rushed all the time, it is unrealistic of nurses to expect them to clear up. 'Anyway, nurses are meant to keep the ward tidy and clear up after doctors, aren't they? Its not really a problem because most doctors tidy up after themselves, like I do' (Appendix N).

Consultants are more likely to see tidying as being part of a nurse's job. But Consultants rarely have to do 'messy' procedures at the bedside; it is to junior doctors that this task tends to fall. Staff Nurses are less likely than Sisters to identify tidying as an area of difficulty. However, as they advance in their career, the continual expectation that they should tidy may become particularly irksome.

'I don't think there is any way of having a policy on

something like that. Its rather like asking who does the washing up. . . .' *Registrar*

'If the nurses are going to abrogate their responsibility for tidying up as well, then one really quite wonders what they are supposed to do.' *Consultant*

'Very often it is seen as a nursing job to clear up. The doctors see themselves as above that, and this is a particular problem with the more junior doctors.' *Senior Registrar*

'To be fair, if the doctor is like really, really mega-busy and you're not, then you don't mind, as long as they don't expect you to do it, you don't mind offering . . . (laughs)' *Sister*

'But if you go in the treatment room when doctors have been there, its like going in the kitchen when your husband's been there, you know that he's been and things are everywhere [laugh], so they cause us work in that sense, they don't seem to believe in tidying up after themselves.' *Staff Nurse*

'But what happens in the end, is usually we nag the doctors and they don't do anything and we end up thinking 'oh well', and clear it up anyway.' *Staff Nurse*

'I don't see why nurses can't clear up. We are supposed to maintain a safe environment, I don't really mind who does it as long as somebody does it. . .' *Staff Nurse*

'If a doctor makes a mess on the trolley and leaves the trolley and abandons it in another room I will bleep them and if they don't come back and clear it up, I will get the Registrar and say that there is bad practice here and if the doctor makes this mess, then he should clear it up.' *Sister*

Particular anger was expressed by some nurses because of the doctors' attitude that nurses ought to tidy up. Like making coffee, the matter is seen as trivial by doctors, but arouses the passion of nurses trying to move away from the handmaiden role of the past. An association between tidying and men's behaviour in the home was made by a few nurses. It is not clear to what extent the gender of nurses plays a role with regard to tidying. Fewer male nurses experienced tidying as a problem. Male nurses appeared to be more likely to resist tidying if they felt it was expected or taken for granted, and male nurses were more likely than female nurses to tell a doctor off or leave them a note. Women doctors were more likely than men to say they tried to tidy up after themselves (56% of women compared with 37% of men). However, no mention of any difference in the behaviour of male and female doctors was made by nurses.

## Tidying and gender

Nurses' resistance to doctors' expectations that nurses should tidy may be linked to gender. Yet many nurses do, and are happy to, tidy up after doctors, both male and female. Many nurses do feel that it is their job to 'maintain a safe environment' for patients. It is also accepted practice to tidy trolleys which doctors have used when carrying out a procedure. If nurses are to hand when a doctor does make a mess, it is accepted that the nurse will tidy. To this extent, nurses do act as the hand maids of doctors.

There are many reasons for nurses to tidy, not least of which is the fact that nurses have to live with the mess on the ward. Whether the mess be needles left on a patient's bed, patients' notes left out, trolleys to be cleared away or coffee cups to be collected, it is the nurse who sees the mess. It is the nurse who knows that visitors, whether patients' relatives or Consultants, to the ward will also see that mess and ascribe it to lackadaisical nurses. The cleanliness of a ward and its apple-pie order was used as a benchmark for the quality of nursing in the recent past. A neatness and tidiness are still seen as the hallmarks of an efficient and well-run ward. It is difficult for nurses to live with a mess, therefore, they tidy the mess up. Doctors, in going to another ward, can leave the mess. Doctors are not being evaluated by the state of the ward.

In considering the issue of tidying, it seems that gender may be less influential than the other differences in status, power, knowledge, class. These findings need further investigation. Tidying seems to act as a barometer with regard to inter-professional relationships. Further research would be rewarding.

Nurses' irritations and resentments about tidying were associated with the view that doctors often cause them more work than necessary. Having to remind doctors about tasks which hadn't been done, or being asked to do things that weren't their job, were moans quite often voiced by nurses. Yet doctors also felt that nurses caused them work by pestering them or calling them unnecessarily. Leaving nurses with tidying up to do may have been an expression of frustration from other areas. The interconnections of all areas of conflict must be borne in mind. In the day-to-day working relations, none is isolated from each other.

## INTRAVENOUS DRUGS

Another area of particular conflict is the issue of the administration of intravenous (IV) drugs. Junior doctors are constantly being reminded to come to the ward to give IVs. They become irritated that nurses can't, or won't, give IV drugs. Why shouldn't nurses give IVs, they're not difficult to give and nurses are there on the ward all the time? Nurses could give IVs as part of their drug rounds. Nurses would reply that they have plenty to do without having to do doctors' tasks as well. Part of the difficulty here is that nurses need to have an 'extended role certificate' which gives them legal cover through the Health Authority for carrying out tasks which are outside normal nursing duties. This certificate enables nurses to administer intravenous drugs (but not the first dose). Nurses who hold the certificate may conceal the fact from their medical colleagues, or they may be unwilling to give IV drugs at all. These nurses may feel they haven't enough time already to give the quality of patient care they would like to give. They may resent doctors' attempt to dump their unwanted tasks onto nurses. Outside specialties such as ITU where nurses routinely give IV drugs, nurses have discretion as to whether or not they give them. The administration of IV drugs is properly the responsibility of doctors. Generally, however, whether or not a junior doctor will be called to administer IV drugs depends, to some extent, on the attitudes of the nursing staff to that doctor and to the role of the nurse. Again here, the negative power of nurses can be seen, as can the nurses' ability to make a junior doctor's life miserable.

'Yes, of course it is an area they can do, it is not a thing that requires any brain power at all, all it requires is some muscle action. That's all there is to it.' *Registrar*

'Things like taking blood, giving IV drugs, setting up IV infusions. I mean my personal opinion is that I think that nurses would be a lot better at doing some of the things than the medical staff, but at the moment I think that we have got enough to do. And I wouldn't like to see our role extended any more because I mean the nurses have got more than enough to do with their own job. But I mean there is plenty of doctors that would you know hand over the menial tasks to the nurses.' *Sister*

'The [Senior] Sister has never really encouraged us to do our certificate, although she has got hers, again she tends to ask the doctors to do their own IV drugs and have more contact with the patient. You find that the drugs are evaluated that much quicker and put onto oral medication.' *Sister*

'If you've got to wait for a doctor to get out of bed and gather his senses, before he comes to add something to a bag of fluid, I'd far more rather give it knowing that I'm awake and competent, than a doctor that comes in half asleep, and they could get the wrong drug or anything. I think the patients will benefit from the nurses having extended roles.' *Staff Nurse*

'We have got about 20 IV drugs to do at each drug round and one of the doctors last week we actually asked her if she would help out and do some and she said 'No, it's not my job, it's your job!' At which point we politely refused to do any of them!' *Staff Nurse*

The question of IV drugs is part of a very long-running saga in which certain tasks undertaken by the medical profession are ceded to nursing staff. For example, taking blood pressures is today an accepted part of the nurse's job yet 30 years ago it was performed only by doctors. As some of the comments make clear, doctors see it as a menial job, not requiring particular expertise and which can be done easily by nurses, as long as they have been trained. (Formal training in the giving of IV drugs is not received by doctors.) Doctors' attempts to pass on some of their tasks to nurses have been challenged by nursing through the concept of the extended role. Thus, tasks such as IV drugs are not part of normal nursing duties but are an **extension** of them. The division within the ranks of nurses about taking on such additional tasks will be addressed in Chapter 9. For the moment, however, it is worth noting that nearly half the nurses and most of the doctors feel that nurses should be giving IV drugs (Appendix O).

Perhaps one reason for nurses' willingness to give IVs arises from one of the features of administering antibiotics by intravenous injection. IVs ought to be given at regular intervals, enabling the optimum level to be maintained in the blood stream. If delayed, then the efficacy of the drug may be correspondingly reduced with potentially undesirable effects to the patient.

## COLLEAGUES' EXPECTATIONS

Underpinning these three issues of tidying, the bleep and the administration of IV drugs are contradictory notions about the role of the nurse in relation to that of the doctor. What doctors want is for nurses to use their initiative, but do what they are told; for nurses to be reliable but biddable. And nurses are to be skilled, but not question doctors' decisions. (There are, of course, similarly contradictory expectations from nurses as to the role of the doctor.)

Nurses are being asked simultaneously to use their initiative yet to be happy to undertake menial and time-consuming tasks for the medical profession. The demands for nurses to perform these tasks are not necessarily motivated by a wish of doctors to improve patient care. While the giving of IV drugs by nurses may be in the interest of patients, limiting the amount of calls to a doctor or tidying up after a doctor are not so obviously of benefit to patients. The impetus to shift the division of labour is not from the quality of service, but reflects the operation of numerous underlying influences in the relationships between doctors and nurses.

The medical professions' expectation that nurses should do these tasks reveals the workings of a variety of factors.
**Power**: on the basis of power, it is quite reasonable that the more powerful group should expect the less powerful group to do whatever tasks it deems appropriate.

**Status**: cleaning is not a high-status occupation and therefore should be done by a lower-status occupational group. Similarly, the administration of IV drugs has come to be seen as a task of relatively low status and should, as a result, be carried out by a lower-status group. As a corollary to this, the greater status accorded to Consultants means that they are never asked to tidy up after themselves. Nurses accept Consultants' claims to be exempt from such duties. It is with junior doctors and only at this low rank, that there is a squabble about who is to tidy. A Senior Registrar will not be asked to tidy, a Registrar rarely and a Senior House Officer fairly often. It is the junior House Officer, the grade of doctor who is not fully established in the role of doctor, whose status is questioned and who is repeatedly asked to tidy up after his or her self.

Status differences within nursing will also affect the division of labour. A Senior Ward Sister will not expect or be expected to tidy up after a junior doctor. The Sister will ask a more junior grade of nurse to tidy a mess up. A Senior Sister will, however, be expected to make decisions about calling a junior doctor out at night. And a Senior Sister is much more likely than her junior nurses to be able to administer IV drugs. The way in which status differentials operate are highly constrained by the nature of the tasks, and how they are viewed.

**Class**: it is not appropriate for members of a lower social class to determine the tasks that their superiors will do. Nurses, in asserting that junior doctors ought to tidy up after themselves are trying to move away from roles previously closely associated with nursing. This relatively recent endeavour by some nurses to ensure that junior doctors tidy up after themselves is a rejection of the deferential role that nurses have previously played. Cleaning, for example, has always been seen as a task particularly appropriate for lower class females. The wish of nurses to be seen as equals and/or treated with respect is correspondingly an attempt to move from an inferior position.

**Gender**: nurses do not mention any difference in tidying between male and female doctors. Similar proportions of both the 'honorary' and the 'real men' of medicine expect nurses to tidy up. Is the act of tidying, a low-status job, associated more with gender or with class? We have male street cleaners and female office cleaners. The acceptance that acting as an assistant or working as a facilitator are women's work is endemic in our society. It is women who act as assistants in offices, banks, industrial enterprises. For the most part, women are subordinate to men. As receptionists in doctors' surgeries, as secretaries to managers and directors, women act as filters for their employers or bosses. These 'filtering' roles assume the greater importance of those whose time is precious, and the filterers are those whose time is used in protecting that preciousness. Most managers are men and most bosses are men. It seems an attractive idea that much of the conflict between nurses and doctors is based on gender. Yet male nurses are little different in their perceptions of tidying. Male nurses are slightly less keen to say that nurses should administer IVs and more aware that doctors want to hand over IVs to nurses. Female doctors are more likely to complain about being called and bleeped than male doctors. Yet the differences here as elsewhere are not great, and it is not obvious that gender is playing a substantial role in the perceptions of the divisions of labour. It seems likely that the operation of class, status, and power is more influential in expectations about the division of labour than the gender of the workforce. It will be interesting to monitor the division of labour as the number of women doctors working in hospitals increase in line with their growing presence in medical schools. For the moment, however, gender appears to be less influential than professional power and status.

**Professional power**: there is the operation of, and the wish to maintain, professional power and the accompanying need to rebuff the advances of an aspiring profession. As medical techniques increase in sophistication and complexity, there is a need for the profession to divest itself of some of its more onerous and less-prestigious tasks. The tasks that are seen as more, or less, prestigious change over time, being affected by a variety of factors, too numerous to go into here. The way in which tasks are moved from one occupational group to another is intriguing. The tasks needs to be 'sold' as something worth doing. Giving IVs is part of the 'extended' role of the nurse. This implies that nurses are being called to enlarge their sphere of competence, to extend themselves. The same task which is to extend nurses is, in reality, being sloughed off by doctors. The routine and time-consuming nature of the task is played down by emphasising the importance of regular administration of IV drugs which nurses can provide. It is worth noting that only a small minority of doctors mentioned the benefits to patients of regularly administered IV drugs. One nurse mentioned the benefits to patients in doctors giving IV drugs, in that they would have greater contact with patients.

**Territorial base**: the ward-based nurse, as mentioned above, has to live with any mess left by a doctor or to tidy it up. The hospital-based doctor can leave it. The ward-based nurse is in a position to more easily administer IV drugs at regular intervals. The nurse has no 'travelling time' between wards to consider, and has no claims to her attention in other locations. By virtue of her presence, the nurse cannot overlook the need for IVs to be given. By her continuing presence, the nurse will also be less able to resist pressures to take over the administration of IV drugs.

**Numbers**: the relative scarcity of doctors and apparent abundance of nurses is another factor affecting who does what. Greater value is attached to scarce commodities than those which are in abundance. Nurses have traditionally been treated as a disposable workforce (Mackay, 1989, p.92) and one that is not highly valued within the NHS. On the other hand, members of a scarce and therefore valued occupation like medicine have to be nurtured and protected. Associated with the differing numbers of nurses and doctors are the economic arguments. It makes sense in an era where cost reduction is all important to ensure that the less-well paid group takes on tasks from the better-paid group. Calls to reduce junior doctors' hours will ensure increased pressure on nurses to take over doctors' tasks. In theory the argument is sound but in practice, doctors will assert the growing demands on their time which result from technological developments in medicine. In turn, there will be no reduction in the numbers of doctors. Similarly, nurses are likely to be asked to do more work in the same amount of time with the same amount of nurses.

**Roles**: the roles to which doctors and nurses aspire affect the division of labour. Doctors as life-savers should not be asked or expected to do tasks which less influential occupations can perform. The special respect given to those who can fight death and prolong life is another reason for the ability of doctors to reject particular tasks. Thus, it is below the dignity and position of doctors to tidy. It is a task which contaminates their claims to superiority over nurses.

There are so many factors which affect the perception of the division of labour between occupations. Different factors will assume primacy at different times. There will be an interplay between these aspects ensuring that it is difficult to untangle the web of influences at any one moment in time. An overarching theory trying to explain the division of labour needs to take account of too many variables to be of any predictive or usable value.

Other areas of responsibility are presently under negotiation: such as wound dressings, taking blood samples, doing ECGs, admitting patients, prescribing drugs. The debates will be parried back and forth between the two occupations. There is little doubt about the longer-term outcome: the dominant profession is likely to remain dominant by virtue of its superior status, power, class, academic requirements, etc. However, the extent to which nursing (or other health care occupations) can whittle away some of that dominance is less clear.

There is now another 'joker' in the pack. The recent changes in the NHS: hospital trusts, internal markets, GP budgets, and a burgeoning private sector, are underlining the importance of costs. Governments' assaults on the professions will continue and none will be more successful than that guided by money. Nurses and doctors will not be able to maintain their running battle over the division of labour: it will be resolved by comparisons of costs. In these terms, the attempt must be made to delegate more and more tasks to the lowest paid. In future, less and less reliance must be placed on the highly skilled because they are expensive and in short supply. This will affect not only the division of labour between doctor and nurse, but also that between qualified and unqualified nurse.

Conflict between occupations is inevitable and natural. As will be seen in Chapter 6, it can be beneficial for the patients and for the delivery of a reflective health care service. The consideration of conflict also illustrates the difficulty in overcoming it. Although attempts can be made to minimize conflict, given the convoluted influences involved in its generation, those attempts are unlikely to be particularly successful.

# 6

# Where it hurts: caring for the dying

Dead patients don't tell tales. They can't tell you what it was like to die or how they were treated. Their relatives and friends can perhaps tell you something about the dying of that patient, but they are not there all the time. Because the patient dies, there are no witnesses to the way that the dying are dealt with. For this reason, the way in which the dying are cared for is particularly important. It is bad enough being an 'outsider' in hospitals. Being uncared for, or insufficiently cared for, when you are dying is the ultimate indignity.

Great care and assiduous attention need to be paid to the most vulnerable of patients. Dying is a lonely business and the dying need friends. But what are friends for? To ensure that your life is as long as possible? To ensure that you end your life with some dignity and peace? To ensure that you experience as little pain as possible? To ensure that all that can be done, is done for you? To ensure that you get the best possible care? Some of these aims are mutually exclusive for the dying person. Choices have to be made as to how a dying patient is to be treated. Indeed, decisions must be made as to when someone is designated as 'dying'. The whole area of dealing with patients who are dying is fraught with difficult decisions and unanswerable questions. It is also an area in which there is considerable dispute between doctors and nurses. The presence of dispute and conflict between nurses and doctors should be welcomed, if it means that decisions regarding the dying patient are well-considered and reflected upon. It is the absence of such conflict which should give cause for concern and suspicion.

## WHEN SHOULD TREATMENT BE STOPPED?

Not surprisingly, conflicts related to the care of the dying
patient and in particular when to stop 'active treatment' of
patients can involve passionate outbursts and considerable
heart-searching. Runciman (1983, p.95) in a study of Ward
Sisters also noted the 'real distress' involved in the disagreements with medical staff about 'the care of the terminally ill,
the management of pain and relief of symptoms, and the care
and resuscitation of elderly patients.' It is an area in which
there are few rules and fewer easy decisions.

> 'A couple of times it's caused a lot of angry tension between
> us . . . here was a patient who'd had life-saving treatment,
> which later failed, but like a year later. It was gradually
> happening, the medical staff couldn't see that they weren't
> treating her with humanity. They couldn't accept that they'd
> failed on this patient, and the patient herself was a very,
> very difficult person and . . . however much you . . . she
> made us feel that we weren't doing enough for her . . . we
> knew it wasn't us, and . . . they wouldn't listen to us, I
> wasn't actually here in the final stages but . . . it was
> dreadful I gather.' *Staff Nurse*

> 'What comes across is doctors are going to treat the patient
> by the book to the bitter end, and I've seen some dreadful
> things in this hospital, things that I cannot forgive . . . I've
> seen a patient die screaming, and it's extremely harrowing
> to see that, and the doctors refuse to give any analgesia or
> whatever. That I cannot forgive, because as one Registrar
> said, 'oh, it's only a certain oedema', this woman lay
> screaming for 12 hours, 24 hours, I mean, the whole ward
> was complaining because she was keeping them awake –
> she was in a cubicle – because the Registrar is afraid of his
> boss. A lot of that goes on. I cannot forgive that.' *Staff Nurse*

> 'We had a six-year-old that was with us for about 5 weeks,
> having chemotherapy, and we know . . . that this girl was
> obviously going to be another one – at one point there was
> almost an open row about it on the unit. Everybody just
> wanted the doctors to withdraw and unfortunately by the
> time that it was accepted, it was too late for the parents who
> just couldn't cope with it and they just walked away from

the situation and therefore didn't have the chance to see the end.' *Staff Nurse*

'Yes, I have known it in special care that nurses are very unhappy about not continuing care even though doctors feel that this child has an extremely poor future, and that further supportive care may be not in that baby's or that baby's family's interest.' *Senior Registrar*

'. . .maybe an elderly patient that they pull out all stops to take them into theatre and do all kinds of horrendous operations, and at the end of the day there's very little result from it. And I think that probably sometimes we would be more likely to say 'well 86 years old is it worth doing an oesophageal transection or something on them, why not just . . . .' *Staff Nurse*

'I have from time to time seen my junior people engaged in resuscitating a patient, or trying to resuscitate a patient, who I would have thought in my own judgment they should never have been started. But you must always respect the fact that they act according to their instincts, and according to what they think is the right thing to do at the time, and I think that you have to accept that obviously.' *Consultant*

Decisions which have to be made about dying patients centre around a number of aspects:

1. When to stop using antibiotics which are putting off an inevitable and imminent death.
2. When to increase the dosage of pain-killing drugs which simultaneously are likely to hasten the death of the patient.
3. When to switch off ventilators which are keeping a patient artificially alive.
4. When to stop undertaking investigative procedures which, while they may help medical research, are doing nothing (or even positive harm) to the terminally ill patient.
5. Decisions regarding chemotherapy and radiotherapy which may be given as a last-hope therapy with little chance of success at considerable cost in patient discomfort and pain through side-effects.

6. Whether or not to make an attempt to resuscitate a patient as, for example, following a cardiac arrest.

## CAUSES OF CONFLICT

Conflicts or difficulties regarding treatment of the terminally ill patients were mentioned quite frequently. Over one-fifth of the doctors and nurses specifically mentioned problems in this area. The various other questions about getting angry, irritations, and mutterings, elicited many further examples of differences of opinion in the treatment of dying patients. In three of the locations nurses and doctors were specifically asked about decisions regarding the treatment of the terminally ill (Appendix P). Just over one-quarter of the doctors and just under one-third of the nurses said there was no problem regarding these treatment decisions. Over two-thirds of the doctors and over half of the nurses said there were occasions on which conflicts occurred. The severity of this conflict varied. For some, there were vividly-remembered incidents while for others, there was resignation regarding the inevitability that there would be differences of opinion. (It was Senior House Officers, Sisters and Registrars who were most likely to report that conflict regarding the treatment of the terminally ill had occurred.)

The more 'aggressive' treatment undertaken by medical staff in teaching hospitals was mentioned by a number of senior doctors and may exert a particularly strong impact on the amount of conflict. Particularly aggressive treatment may be undertaken for a number of reasons such as research, to try out new treatment or to get 'good figures' for the regular audit of patient deaths.

'In that case the senior doctor said 'well obviously this patient's not going to die' and everyone else had come to the conclusion the patient was going to die and wanted him to die as nicely as possible. And he decided just because it had been a surgical ward and he'd had a bad spate and a lot of people had actually died that week, none were his fault, but they had died and it was going to look bad on the audit thing – you know all these people are presented as dying at the audit. I think he decided he sort of wanted to stop this sort of flow for a wee minute.' *Senior House Officer*

## Decision making

The responsibility for making decisions in the treatment of terminally ill patients varies from one situation to another. Decision-making is the responsibility of doctors, but information will be offered by, or sought from, nurses. Joint decisions by nurses and doctors will also be made, but the decision remains the final responsibility of doctors. Who actually takes the decision depends on the circumstances: the doctor who is in control in the arrest situation will take the decision not to continue with attempts to resuscitate. When to stop active treatment, by say withdrawing antibiotic drugs, is a decision taken by Consultants and, in their absence from the ward, by Registrars. Instigating diamorphine infusion is a decision often taken by Senior House Officers. As the on-call doctors, SHOs will be placed in the situation of decision-making during the night and will have to respond to, say, nursing requests to make the patient pain-free. Decisions to take patients off a ventilator tend to be made by Consultants. In all these areas, decisions can be, and are taken by, different grades of doctors. Even although a Consultant may have made a decision to 'keep on going' with a particular patient, junior doctors and nursing staff may themselves quietly agree to 'let the patient go'.

### Seeking opinion

Whichever grade of doctor takes the final decision, those who directly care for that patient ought to be consulted in order to obtain up-to-date information regarding the patient and the wishes of the relatives. It is here that the claim that nurses spend a great deal of their time with patients can be shown to be exaggerated. It is student nurses, unqualified nursing staff and domestics who are most likely to be in contact with the dying patient (Mills, 1983; Field, 1989). Greater recognition needs to be given to this aspect. Qualified nurses may well shun the dying patient, especially when medical treatment has been withdrawn. However, there can be a marked contrast in

ITU areas, where the critically ill patient can soon become the dying patient. In intensive therapy, highly technical nursing needs to be combined with the special care required by relatives of dying patients.

Auxiliary nurses often have particular knowledge of patients and indeed, may have greater contact than the qualified nursing staff. It is to auxiliaries that patients or their relatives may be most confiding, yet the possibility of including auxiliaries in decisions such as terminating care seem to be seldom considered. Domestic staff and nursing auxiliaries have little contact with doctors and are, therefore, less influenced by the medical model of care. They are likely to have a perspective substantially different from that of doctors, and some nurses. It is seldom the doctor who holds the hand of the dying patient. Yet such a demanding role falls to those who are not asked for their opinions as to the appropriate treatment for the patient. Of course, if information is not sought from those 'at the bedside' there is much less possibility of conflicting views being presented and decisions are easier to make. The moral and emotional dilemmas can, in this way, be minimized. At the same time, doctors are schooled to think that they and only they 'know best'.

Similarly, the maintenance of status differences seems to be more important for doctors than obtaining as much information as possible. Not only are auxiliary nurses not consulted, even nursing staff may sometimes not be asked for their opinion. Doctors enjoy being able to count on the judgement of nurses, yet the ability of nurses to have special and particular knowledge of a patient is not always apparent in the responses to questions regarding the care of the terminally ill. Although quite a number of nurses report that their opinions are listened to in the care of the terminally ill, it seems that those opinions are often not heeded. Listening but not hearing the opinions of nurses appears to be a particular source of difficulties in the care of the terminally ill.

### Dealing with relatives

Dealing with relatives is a substantial part of caring for the dying. It is to qualified nurses that dealing with relatives normally falls. Indeed, speaking to relatives seems to be one of the activities which doctors are only too pleased to hand over to nurses. It can be an onerous task: emotionally demanding as well as being time consuming. What comfort can be given to a wife when her husband is dying, or to a father when his child is diagnosed as having cancer? Nurses may not actually break the bad news to relatives, but they will have the repeated contact with relatives which doctors may not have.

'Its like tonight I've got in. . . . I'm looking after a poorly boy whose Mum and Dad were sat here. And one of the other nurses said that all weekend, they hadn't been involved in his care. Well if I've got somebody like that, I like them to – if they want to – then they look after that . . . so they've washed him, changed him, changed the sheets and they went away a lot happier tonight, they've actually been involved. That's different nursing care rather than doctor. . . .' *Sister*

In this case, the nurse was able and willing to identify the needs of relatives and to make room for those. Too often the hidden demands for nursing care can be overlooked if attention is paid solely to medical aspects of care and treatment.

## Nurse and doctor involvement

The presence of some conflict in making decisions about the treatment of the terminally ill is, in theory, good. It means that differing views of the patient and of health care have been presented and come up for debate. It also means that decisions are taken in the light of all the immediately available information. In practice, the conflict that occurs is often because a course of action is being pursued by the medical staff in the absence of any nursing input regarding the patient's condition. As Elston (1977b, p.29) notes, the medical profession perceives greater danger in non-treatment than over-treatment. Nurses do not find it easy to question doctors' decisions. When disagreement is expressed, it tends to erupt and be full of anger and frustration rather than clearly reasoned argument. The focus of dispute moves from the patient to inter-professional relations. Too easily, therefore, occupational fighting can replace concern for the patient.

Nurses and doctors will have personal preferences and one person's 'bad' patient is another person's 'good' patient. There are patients with whom there is an immediate rapport and empathy. The possibility of such a rapport is greater in the longer-stay specialties, both for doctors and nurses. The possibility of such a rapport is greater for nurses than for doctors. In specialties such as intensive care, nurses will have an intense involvement with many of the patients for whom they care. The importance of each patient is implicit in the attention they receive. For a nurse to spend a number of days giving total patient care to one person almost inevitably means some emotional bond with that patient. Intensive care is known to be one of the most stressful specialties in which to nurse. Many patients die and some of them take time in their dying. There is particular stress in nursing patients who are in great discomfort. There is particular stress in nursing the brain-dead (Allan, 1989). The close monitoring of patients means that the nurse is highly attuned to slight changes in the patient's condition. The intensive care nurse, highly trained and with specialist skills, is likely to have both a subjective and objective relationship with her patient. Difficulties with the decisions as to when to stop active treatment are often mentioned by nurses in intensive care, yet such nurses are more likely to feel that their opinions are listened to, and acted upon, by their medical colleagues. The conflict seems to emerge when doctors from specialties other than ITU/ anaesthetics are the 'owners' of patients. These 'outside' doctors are sometimes loathe to give up on patients and may make last-ditch attempts to save them. The nurses, with their experience and knowledge of patients and the emotional state of the relatives, may feel particularly aggrieved that they are not asked their opinion regarding patient management of the terminally ill.

> 'You notice very much that some Consultants are very much more unwilling to sort of give up than others. And that's upsetting for the nurses, I think it must be awful, and I've seen people lying and you think my God why don't they just die, why don't we just let them die, at least I only see them when I am walking past sort of thing, whereas the

nurses they are the ones that have to look at it all the time, I think that must be very upsetting for them.' *House Officer*

'I think I can identify their particular group of patients which causes us all a lot of heartache and they are patients who really are terminally ill, who haven't responded to the appropriate treatment, but the owners (the admitting Consultants) aren't prepared to discontinue.' *Consultant Anaesthetist*

'I think that looking after patients just on this unit alone, that you know are going to die, but the doctors won't . . . aren't prepared to stop treating until they've gone through absolutely everything, even though they know that they are going to die as well, they are not prepared to stop treating. I think that's very, very stressful, 'cause you are . . . well not for the patient, 'cause very often they are out of it by that stage, but for relatives it's very distressing for the relatives, because every time they come in they see a new drip, or a new piece of equipment they think there's hope, and really you know in your heart that there isn't hope, and the doctor knows that as well if he's being honest, but. . .' *Staff Nurse*

## How to decide

There is a conflict between the perspectives of nurses and doctors regarding the treatment of the terminally ill (Runciman, 1983, p.96). Nurses tend to be more concerned with the kind of death that patients have and whether it is peaceful, pain-free and dignified. The more passive, consoling role of the nurse does little to fight death but accepts it as part of life. Our Western cultures' fear of death is part of the reason for the ascendancy of the medical profession in our lives and for our willingness to accept the medicalization of society. Doctors, because they are responsible for life and death decisions, have to ensure that they have done all they can. Doctors must shun the easy option of saying 'full nursing care' for as long as they can. They feel they have a duty to do so. Doctors are only too aware that their action or inaction can have irrevocable consequences. Nurses, who are not in the same unenviable position, can advance their views in the safe knowledge that the responsibilities of the doctor will act as a balance to their perspective.

'The sort of medical ethic is that patients live as long as you can possibly carry it on. If they die it's your failure, and there's an awful lot of that feeling, particularly among surgeons and physicians, other specialties aren't quite so bad, but wanting to treat somebody with intravenous antibiotics or just some other form of treatment which is in fact, expensive and its not actually doing the patients any good or making them more comfortable. It's going to prolong their life inappropriately. And quite often it's sort of a moral decision that I actually get very cross about.' *Sister*

Nevertheless, life-prolonging action needs to be taken with as much thought as life-shortening action. Many nurses would like doctors to more closely examine their reasons for keeping a patient alive. Nurses have suggested that doctors do so because they hate to admit their failure. To some doctors, it seems as though medicine is a fight with death and a fight to control death. 'Giving up' on a patient is not only admitting failure – it can also result in feelings of guilt and of doing less than one's best.

'You have taken an oath that you are going to help people, and . . . I can't go through the whole oath but basically active euthanasia doesn't come into it, although providing analgesia at a level sufficient to keep the patients pain free and undistressed is part of caring for them. Turning a diamorphine pump up so that they die quicker than they could be isn't.' *House Officer*

'I think that you have got to let your patient die with dignity, whereas a lot of doctors, perhaps more junior, feel that if they lose somebody they are wrong, it is something they have done, and I think that they forget that we have got to allow people to die with dignity, and death is a big part of our job.' *Sister*

'But sometimes you say "no, you know, we have done everything we can and this patient is going to die within the next few hours, or certainly in the next day or two", and at that point I feel that the nursing and medical staff have a responsibility not to prolong death. You know some people would say that's playing God, think that the actual act of prolonging death is playing God. When death is inevitable it really should be made as dignified as possible, and I think that . . . I mean there has been a change, and I think that we are much more willing to admit this now.' *Consultant*

'I would say that everybody is uneasy about making the decisions although we know deep inside what should happen. I think that nobody wants to be the person to come out and actually say it or do it, I think.' *Staff Nurse*

'Doctors in the main try not to get too close to their patients, because too many of them over the years probably die, have problems, if you got involved in every one of their problems, as an intensive care doctor you have a very high death rate, or if you are a doctor covering a resuscitation area, you probably couldn't function.' *Senior Registrar*

### When to decide

Another difficulty in the care of the terminally ill is the unpredictability of illness. The certainty of medical knowledge is always open to question. Decisions to stop active treatment too early can be wrong. But how are doctors to know when 'too early' is? Doctors must play for time in order to achieve greater certainty in the correctness of their decision-making. Certainly in one case recounted to us, the decision to stop active treatment was a life-saver. The slightly misplaced sense of humour of the nurse had made this Consultant rather angry:

'Once, fairly recently as it happens, yes, I can distinctly remember a nurse rather lightheartedly suggesting that – this was a particular patient, who, rather unexpectedly, got better, I mean, we'd wholly expected the patient to die, and we'd withdrawn treatment – and she suggested that we should stop our treatments more often, perhaps we'd get more patients alive, but that wasn't the only remark, there were one or two others, which of course were meant as jokes, but, I think, rather sick jokes.' *Consultant*

The uncertainty of medical knowledge gives additional

stress in the management of patients who are terminally ill. That uncertainty is not often acknowledged. Indeed, it almost cannot be acknowledged because doctors set great store by the science of medicine. The predictability presupposed in scientific knowledge is contradicted by every physician's experience in which each case is, no matter how little, different. This is not the place to delve further into the basis of medical knowledge. However, the uncertainty of outcome of medical decision-making acts as one of the strong reasons for trying everything possible and not acting too hastily. There is no doubt of the difficulty about the dilemmas involved in the care of the terminally ill. It is junior doctors who are most likely to find greatest difficulty in dealing with the terminally ill. For these junior doctors, medicine is likely to appear more powerful and stronger than it really is. They may be less philosophical that their older colleagues who have learned to accept 'failures'. The newly-qualified junior doctor is also more likely to have established a relationship with a patient with a corresponding emotional tie. And in this way junior doctors can feel personally responsible for 'giving up' on a patient and feel they themselves are 'letting the patient down'. Of course, whether or not death is seen as a failure is in part dependent on the specialty in which the doctor is working (Field, 1989, p.64). The guilt accompanying 'the failure' to save a patient which doctors can experience is appreciated by some nurses:

> 'Basically I always used to try and get everybody behind me so it's not just me thinking that. I make sure that the doctor won't feel guilty . . . and usually anyway I find . . . erm . . . the Consultants, because they've been doing care of the elderly for so long, they really understand, and you know, you don't always have to ask them, but if you did, then they would definitely come down and say no, we'll call it a day . . . and that will give the doctors more strength to say, right well we won't treat any more . . . because it must be difficult for them, to make that decision.' *Sister*

For a patient you have come to know well, it is undoubtedly difficult to stop 'fighting' on that patient's behalf and accepting the inevitable. Nurses are quite aware of the difficulties involved in 'giving up' (Field, 1989, p.79). But the greater distance which Consultants maintain from patients perhaps makes decisions about the treatment of the terminally ill easier.

## ASKING RELATIVES' ADVICE

The need to take account of relatives' wishes and fears compounds the difficulties in caring for the terminally ill. In some cases, the patient is not in any state to contribute to any decision regarding his or her care. The burden then moves to the relatives. The inability of a patient's relatives to cope with a lingering and painful death or their wish for everything possible to be done will vitally affect the approach taken. Having to talk to, calm and deal with relatives is a task often left to nurses. It is a difficult task which is both time-consuming and stressful. Not surprisingly, 'the relatives' are often given as one reason for the need to come to a decision regarding the status of the patient and whether active treatment is to stop.

> We're the ones who are supporting the relatives, and that's when we really get angry as nurses, or when I do, when you say to the doctors, I cannot flannel over the relatives any more, we have got to make a decision today, it's not fair saying that this doctor hasn't yet been in, therefore we can't make a decision, they deserve better than that, is what we end up saying. *Sister, ITU*

> 'We try never to put the relative in the position of making the decision because we don't think that is a reasonable thing to do. . . . I think it's a medical decision that needs to be done because it's impossible for people to end up years later thinking, you know, that they took a decision and perhaps it wasn't a right decision. I think it's got to be taken by the medical and nursing staff, in liaison.' *Senior Registrar*

It must not be assumed that nurses always want to 'give up' on a patient before doctors. For one young child who had been on the unit for many weeks, nursing staff were particularly loathe to stop active treatment when the doctors involved felt that the child's quality of life was exceedingly poor. In casualty, other incidents were recounted of nurses being less willing than doctors to abandon attempts at resuscitation. However, in the majority of cases the nurses were less likely to want to continue treatment than doctors. In the main, doctors were keener to continue treatment of the terminally ill patient.*

## SPEAKING UP

Although many of the nurses' implicitly adopted a 'patient's advocate' stance in their comments made about the treatment of the terminally ill, no explicit mention of this role was made. This is an interesting omission, as some members of the professionalising sector within nursing (which Melia, 1987, p.166, locates in the sphere of nurse education rather than nursing practice) have recently stressed the need for nurses to act as the patient's advocate. There seems to be a belief among some nurses that they are somehow on the patient's side (and by extension that doctors somehow are not). Running counter to this view is another aspect of the nurse-doctor relationship which negatively affects the patient, that of loyalty. An accepted part of the nurse's role is to present, at all costs, a confidence in the abilities and expertise of the doctor. For some nurses, the interests of the patient come second to those of the medical profession. A united front has to be displayed for the patient. In the interests of maintaining trust and confidence, nurses may have to disguise their unease about a certain line of treatment in front of patients. It seems that nurses are often hesitant to speak out to doctors about practices of which they disapprove. And as seen Chapter 5, many doctors do not want to hear what nurses have to say, and particularly they do not want to hear nurses' opinions on the management of patients. So when a nurse says that she would 'side' with a doctor, in other words, maintain a loyalty to her colleagues, that loyalty may be at the expense of the patient. It may mean that the patient is inadequately or inappropriately treated. It may mean that the patient is allowed to experience greater pain or undergo an unnecessary test because the nurse is unwilling, or unable, to be heard. It is

---

* Field (1989, p.75) also found that nurses tend to argue for palliative care at an earlier stage than doctors.

to colleagues with whom one has a continuing relationship that loyalty seems to lie, rather than to the vulnerable individual who is 'passing through'.

'If a patient comes to me and complains about a doctor I think I would tend to take the doctor's side. Well, not take the doctor's side, but not agree with the patient, not allow it sort of to go forward.' *Staff Nurse*

Too easily can nurses and doctors 'gang up' on a patient, looking after their own professional interests rather than those of the patient. In closing ranks and keeping the patient uninformed, the potential for the patient to enjoy any power or autonomy is correspondingly diminished (Millman, 1976, p.137). Of course, the loyalty of the nurse to the doctor is only one part of the equation. The loyalty of one doctor to another, or rather the unwillingness to negatively comment on the practices of another doctor, is unlikely to be in the patient's interest. The individual professional's protection of medicine as a whole is at the expense of the patient. This is an aspect which will be revisited in Chapter 11.

Although some nurses undoubtedly do speak out against what they see as being unacceptable practices in the care of the terminally ill, others do not. Quite a number of nurses were concerned simply to do what the senior doctor told them to do. They seemed to have no interest in a patient advocate's role. For these nurses, what was important was to obey the instructions of the doctor. To some extent, such obedience was realistic: there was little or nothing they could do to influence the doctor. For the less assertive nurse, there is little chance of being heard and if heard, of being attended to. These obedient nurses may serve the medical profession but they do not serve the patient.

Junior doctors are also in a position from which they can gain greater knowledge about the patient than can their seniors. Junior doctors, like nurses, have a great deal more patient contact than senior doctors. It is difficult to speak out against a senior doctor's decision. Just as a 'trouble-maker' label can affect a nursing career, it can similarly damage a medical career. The all-important reference can be a passport to a glowing future hospital career. If the Senior Consultant doesn't want to hear about the psychological state of a patient, then the SHO will not volunteer such information. The Consultant, in other words, sets the agenda as to what information is seen as relevant to his decision-making. The hold which the Consultant has on the junior doctor's activities ensures that dissident voices regarding any lapses or misjudgments in the treatment of patients will not be heard. It is more than a pity that there can be a conflict between pursuing the patient's best interests and maintaining career prospects for the junior doctor. It is the junior doctor, after all, who is the doctor best placed to have a particular awareness of the patient's situation. Between junior doctors and nurses there was evidence of some agreement on the treatment of the terminally ill. The disagreements were sometimes between the senior and the junior doctors.

'Sometimes, say in haematology, they'll put out arrest calls on patients which most people would think entirely inappropriate. But there's no aggravation between ourselves and the nursing staff for putting the call out because you know the situation. The Consultant says there should be one, there is one.' *House Officer*

'I feel it's up to the doctors because I don't think that I'm covered really, legally. I mean it's not going to be my signature on the notes that is going to say this patient is not for resuscitation, if they do pass, they'll pass away.' *Staff Nurse*

## Legal responsibilities

The issue of being legally responsible and the threat of being sued loom excessively in the thoughts of nurses. 'Not being legally covered' was often given as a reason for inaction by nurses. Doctors are clearly aware of their legal responsibility: it is an onerous aspect of their work but one which is accepted in return for the autonomy and independence they enjoy. Nurses, however, because of their lack of power are terrified of doing something wrong. The threat of legal action compounds the effects of the over-emphasis on discipline within nursing. It is a perfect way in which to hobble nurses and prevent independence of thought or action.

## SPEAKING ON BEHALF OF THE PATIENT

It is a poor system if there is no voice to speak on behalf of the patients, when they are at their most vulnerable. Doctors and nurses who fail to speak or ensure that an alternative view of patient management is presented to the senior doctor, are failing the patient. They are looking after their own interests, not those of the patient.

Junior doctors, who are likely to have been and are still being schooled in the way of the medical profession are likely to adopt the predominant views of their senior colleagues. Any reluctance to voice different opinions is understandable given that junior doctors' careers, if they are to be successful hospital careers, are in the hands of these same senior colleagues.

Nurses being in a separate hierarchy from doctors are theoretically, more able to counter the ideas of the medical profession. Nurses do have a different view of patients from doctors. Nurses are ward-based, they see more of the patients, they see more of the relatives, and they are in a better position to establish a relationship with patients than their medical colleagues. Doctors tend to view patients clinically, while nurses are more likely to see the patient as a whole person. While the doctor may see the extent of the disease, the nurse may see the demoralized and despondent patient. The patient that brightens up when the Consultant visits the ward, disguises their own response to their illness. Doctors, if they are aware of this 'perking up when the doctor comes' process, will be careful to ensure that nurses' views are sought. Nurses who are aware of this 'putting a good face on' for the Consultant, ought to be prepared for the patient's sake, to speak up on behalf of the patient. It is nurses who occupy the privileged position of being able to gain the confidences and trust of patients; they ought not to abuse that trust.

In the care of the terminally ill, differing views of the patient are required. Indeed, differing views can strengthen the decision which is taken on behalf of the dying patient. The problem is ensuring that these different views are expressed, and heard, as well as informing the decision-making process. Whether those views come from nurses, junior doctors, or auxiliaries, the 'I-can't-hear-what-you-say-because-of-who-you-are' response is inadequate. Terminally ill patients deserve better than that.

### Encountering death

Our culture has a particular fear of death and doctors and nurses are part of that culture. There is harrowing stress involved in dealing with patients who are dying. Patients do not always die 'nicely'. The process of death can be slow and gentle, or it can be rapid and harsh. Nurses, as students, will have had experience of caring for dying patients, of sitting with them and holding their hands as they die. It is when nurses are extremely young that they will have their first contact with death. It is a frightening occurrence and one which many young nurses fear (Birch, 1975, p.54). It is the 'unfair deaths' of children and young adults which cause greatest stress for nurses (Mackay, 1989, p.66). Yet nurses receive inadequate support and encouragement in dealing with dying patients and therefore seek to restrict their involvement with them (Field, 1989, p.28).

Doctors have less contact with the dying than nurses and are also likely to encounter death at a later stage in their training. The doctor is trained to adopt a scientific and objective stance towards patients and not to become involved, since there is no reward in the system for doctors who do become involved with patients. Emotional involvement is costly in personal terms and, anyway, is not expected of doctors. Talking to terminally ill patients is a source of considerable stress for medical students (Firth, 1986, p.1177), yet the teaching they are given in coping with the terminally ill has not been found to be particularly helpful (Field, 1984, p.433). The emphasis in hospital medicine on curing patients and saving lives involves a fight with death. It is not surprising that a large proportion of Consultants have been found 'not to linger' when medical intervention ceases (Mills, 1983, p.254). For when death is winning, the doctor is losing.

### Nursing the dying patient

Mills (1983, p.140) and Field (1989, p.41) have each reported that nursing practices regarding the dying are often inadequate. When medical interventions have been exhausted or unsuccessful, doctors withdraw their attention and nurses spend less time with patients. The perspective adopted by the

Consultant to the terminally ill patient affects the nursing care. Thus Mills (1983, p.145) found that the 'medical practitioner has a pervasive influence on the activity of the nurse.' The ease with which nurses are turned away from the dying patient is disturbing. It seems that the early lessons of obeying and pleasing others cannot be overcome by nurses. What Sister wants may come before what the patients need (Bond and Bond, 1980, p.27), and nurses are expected to do what doctors want first and what patients want a poor second (Chapman, 1977, p.167).

The patient who is dying is often alone. Mills (1983, p.139) has reported that dying patients were alone for 70–90% of the time, yet the patients were likely to be both conscious and aware of their environment. Mills (1983, p.140) also found that these dying patients were visited less often by nursing staff and were unable to attract the attention of the nurse. When the Consultant expressed interest in the patient, then nurses themselves showed greater interest in the patient. Nurses' interest and involvement with the patient depended on doctors' interest and involvement. Yet Uprichard (1971, p.232) indicates that, 'the relief of the patient's pain, fear, guilt, anxiety, loneliness, grief, etc. is the core of all nursing – whatever the medical diagnosis may be.' It is particularly disappointing that nurses take their lead from the medical profession in this way. It is more than a disappointment to the dying patient desperate for a drink of water and who cannot get their attention: a particularly harrowing example given by Mills (1983).

## THE DEFERENCE OF NURSES TO DOCTORS

Why do some nurses reflect the priorities of the medical profession, rather than those of nursing? In objective terms, as was outlined in Chapter 3, nurses and doctors are not equal. Accompanying the disparities in power, pay, status, etc. is the 'subservience' of nurses to members, and especially to senior members, of the medical profession (Kalisch and Kalisch, 1977, p.53). Nurses, it is argued, have been socialized into subservience (Jolley, 1989) and initiated into submission from their earliest years (Strong and Robinson, 1990, p.38). Nurse training, the organizational structure of the hospital, the structure and practices within the ranks of nursing have variously played a part in perpetuating the subservient relationship of nursing to medicine. The subservience of nurses to doctors is not simply an individual response, but is built into the provision of health care in the UK. Whether in the hospital or the community, nurses are in a subservient position to doctors, a subservience which becomes visible in the deference accorded to doctors by nurses.

Deference is not simply behaviour or attitudes, but a form of social interaction (Newby, 1975, p.146). The structures within which nurses and doctors work ensure that a deferential relationship is perpetuated. The ward round is a good example. The nurse in charge holds the patients' notes for the doctor; when asked, she will offer perhaps a few words about the patient for the doctor's consideration, she prepares the patient for examination and is silent as he examines the patient and decides what action is to be taken. The nurse gives a reassuring smile to the patient and moves with the doctor to the next patient. It is a structured interaction which emphasizes the power and the relationship between the nurse, the doctor and the patient. The formality of the ward round also acts to protect the doctor from the potential stress of close contact with patients.

A deferential relationship is more likely to be found where there is an identifiable local territory giving 'a solidarity of place, to both superordinates and subordinates alike' (Newby, 1975, p.157). Thus in two of the district hospitals visited where greater reliance was made on a local nursing labour force, there was a greater sense of belonging and evidence of a stronger allegiance to doctors by nurses. The more deferential stance adopted by nurses in the Scottish district hospital partly reflected its easily-identified territorial location. Somewhat revealingly, nurses in Scotland made fewer comments about differences of opinion with regard to the treatment of the terminally ill than their English counterparts.

The deference of nurses (among others working in health care) to doctors and the medical profession as a whole is understandable. It is, after all, the medical profession which has set the agenda for the organization and priorities within hospital health care. It is for the attention of the medical profession that patients enter hospitals. Nurses are, to that extent, playing in 'bit parts'. Such a view does not reflect the reality of the care that is given to patients. For example, in the care of the elderly there is relatively little input from the medical profession and an extremely high input from nursing. In psychiatry, the intermittent visits by doctors in which they announce both entry and discharges from the system, are almost incidental to the daily experiences of the patients who spend their days in the care of nurses. The specialties in which there is less medical input and less medical intervention are those specialties which enjoy least status in the hospital pecking order. The status ascribed to hospital specialties by nurses mirrors those of the medical profession (Mackay, 1989; Melia, 1987). Thus, nurses accept the agenda and the pecking order established by the medical profession. In so doing, nurses cement their deferential relationship to the medical profession. (Although it must be said that many nurses actively seek to work in specialties which the medical profession does not highly regard and which offer particular challenges and rewards to nurses.)

Unable to develop a confidence which their training has squeezed out of them, nurses find it hard to speak up. Nurses seek the approval of doctors rather than a development and realization of their own potential (Kalisch and Kalisch, 1977, p.53). The structures into which deference and subservience are built mean that the medical profession's priorities come before those of nurses and patients. Thus the dominance of doctors and of 'the medical model' of health care is part of the reason for nurses' failure to offer sufficient care and attention to the dying.

The deferential stance adopted by many nurses (as opposed to the structures which underpin a deferential relationship) may be particularly inappropriate. Some Consultants said they did not seek deference, although others made clear the fineness of the line between unwelcome deference and insolence! Such a stance is not sought by Consultants. It seems that Consultants respond 'positively to the qualified nurses who demonstrated professional autonomy' (Mills, 1983, p.255–6). It is nurses who ensure that the dominant voice prevails; it is nurses who are compounding the influence of the medical profession. More nurses must voice their own views and not avoid the confrontation that may await their challenge to the views of the medical profession. Their deferential stance does little for the patient. Mills (1983, p.106) reports that only 15.5% of nurses showed characteristics of 'caring' for the dying patient. The remainder treated patients as 'socially dead'. These are shocking figures; this is no way to treat the dying.

# 7

# Perfect partners

'I don't like the phrase "working as a team" because teams usually play **against** someone else and in health care I know jolly well who that is.' (*Katherine Whitehorn, cited by Duncan, 1984, p.88*)

Questions may be asked about the extent to which nurses and doctors put their own occupational interests before those of the patients. However, there is an acceptance that doctors and nurses *ought* to work together, to work collaboratively and cooperatively to maximize the quality of care given to patients.

## 'IDEAL' COLLEAGUES

So how can collaboration between two such disparate occupational groups be achieved? Perhaps if they could change one another, get them to understand and appreciate the stresses and strains of their colleagues? It would be marvellous if we could all have designer-made colleagues to work with. Our working life would be wonderful. All the squabbles and irritations would be ended. We wouldn't use up all our time and energy in having to defend ourselves against colleagues. How would nurses and doctors describe their perfect colleague? What is their ideal of a good nurse or a good doctor like?

The picture of the ideal colleague is built up from a number of different sources. From earliest childhood, ideas are formed about doctors and nurses which will play some part in the decision to enter medicine and nursing. The attributes valued by nurses and doctors will reflect their socialization before they enter the occupation and their socialization within it.

Through the formal training and the informal contacts, the explicit and implicit messages as to the good doctor or the good nurse are received and evaluated. Images of role models follow nurses and doctors through their working lives. The way a certain Sister had her finger on the pulse of everything happening in the ward, or the way that a particular doctor took care to explain the planned treatment to a patient, act as guides to later action.

Each person's view of what constitutes a good nurse or doctor will reflect their own experiences: people they have worked with, people they have heard of, or watched on television. One of the strongest influences on individuals views of the ideal colleague will be their experiences during training. The socialization that takes place during training ensures that the views of the newcomers soon come to reflect those of older colleagues.*

With surprising rapidity the views of nursing students reflect the views of older colleagues (Mackay, 1989). What are the 'ideal types' which are built up by doctors and nurses?

'Ideal types' are composite pictures and do not distinguish between one grade of doctor or nurse and another. Neither do they tend to distinguish between the attributes required in different specialties. Some will be speaking of Sisters, some of House Officers, a few of Consultants. 'Ideals' are 'ideals' and they exist in imagination, not in reality. We might not want to meet them or work with anyone like them: they would be too good to be true. Perfect people can be constant reminders of our own imperfections.

Nevertheless, the idea of a 'good nurse' and a 'good doctor' is implicit in many of the expressed opinions and attitudes of doctors and nurses. The 'ideals' serve as a benchmark against which colleagues' behaviour at work is measured (Bates, 1966a,b).

## THE GOOD NURSE

### The nurse's view

For nurses, the 'good nurse' is caring and sensitive to the needs of patients. She will be thoughtful and attentive. The aspects emphasized by nurses centre on the way a nurse

* For a discussion of the socialization of nurses, refer to Conway (1983). For a personal view of the socialization of a doctor, refer to Marinker (1974).

relates to her patients: the need to be genuine, understanding, patient, kind. The good nurse will listen and communicate well. She will be approachable and she will have time to talk. At the same time she needs to be assertive and remain calm whatever the circumstances. The good nurse doesn't panic, everything is always 'under control'. The patients will trust such a nurse and feel confident when she is around.

'I think first of all you definitely have to be dedicated, sympathetic, obviously you've got to have good practical skills, good bedside manner, good communicator. You've got to look professional, good attitude to behaviour, always have a smiling face even though some things might repulse you, or if you feel ill you've still got to put on a brave face, and just generally do the most that you can for the patient.' *Staff Nurse*

'You can never have a perfect nurse but you can have a nurse who is extremely caring. I think if the nurse does to her patient what she would like done to herself, and be treated as she would like herself to be treated and I think if any nurse keeps that in her mind, then they are pretty damned good. Be able to listen and not dictate.' *Sister*

The good nurse is a good person and especially, a good woman (Gamarnikow, 1978). Nurses' descriptions of her emphasize her personal characteristics. While such attributes can be developed they cannot be learned (Gamarnikow, 1978). This good nurse is born, not made. No matter what training she receives, the special attributes which nurses need cannot be taught. This view of nurses has a long tradition, dating back to Florence Nightingale, who laid great stress on the importance of personal character rather than training or skills (Baly, 1986). For her, the good nurse was quiet, kind and compassionate.*

Few patients would dissent from this view of the good nurse. But there is a curious lack of emphasis on the skills and expertise of nurses. What nurses' do, it seems, is what women

---

* For discussions of the dynamics affecting the image of the nurse, refer to Ehrenreich and English (1973); Kalisch and Kalisch (1986); Salvage (1985).

naturally do and what any mother would do for her child. Clean up their vomit without chastising; be a shoulder to cry on without judging; comfort them when they are in pain or frightened. The need for nurses to have an informed and experienced 'eye' or the need to exercise judgements as to when to take or not to take action, is hardly mentioned. Academic or knowledge of theory is very much of secondary importance, it has little to offer at the bedside. What is of central importance is practical experience and practical skills. In other words, because the good nurse cannot be 'made', the value set upon training and the development of theoretical knowledge is not great. Nurses do not seem to place a high value on their own skills, or on the training they have received (Mackay, 1989).

## The doctor's view

For doctors, the 'good nurse' is first and foremost, competent at her job. She knows about her patients, she can anticipate problems and she will use her initiative. While it is important for a good nurse to be sensitive to the needs of patients, it is even more important for her to act as the doctor's 'eyes and ears' on the ward in his absence. The good nurse can be relied on: she will pick up things that the doctors have missed. She communicates 'well' with doctors: she won't pester them unnecessarily and when she does phone, the doctor knows it must be important. Her judgement can be trusted and the doctor can leave the ward secure in that knowledge when she is on duty.

> 'I think in general, if they're aware of what's going on . . . picking up points that you've missed, because frequently when you're really busy, you do leave things out . . . and I know it's not up to them to keep checking what the doctors are doing, but it's really nice when you've missed something quite obvious, and somebody points it out to you. . . I don't mind it being pointed out to me, I'd like somebody to if I miss something, for goodness sake, please say. . .' *Senior House Officer*

'It is ability to think, to answer, to be inquisitive about problems that are there, an ability to produce solutions or contribute to solutions in relation to managing a patient.'
*Consultant*

The aspect which is of less importance to nurses is of greatest importance to doctors: skill. For doctors, an incompetent nurse is worse than anything. For nurses, an uncaring and unkind nurse is worse than anything.

The competence which doctors value means that a nurse knows when a patient needs attention; she can take decisions; she knows what she's doing, and the ward runs smoothly. Competence also comes through experience and through knowledge. It is an attribute which can be acquired and runs counter to nurses' view that the good nurse is 'born not made'.

It is hardly surprising that doctors emphasize the knowledge and skill aspects, the learned component of work activity. They, after all, have to go through extensive training in which the levels of their knowledge and skill become critical. They have immersed themselves in scientific knowledge at school and at university. Their concern has been with assimilating facts and rejecting feelings. As a glance at any medical school prospectus will show, doctors pride themselves on being scientists. Older views of the intending medical practitioner as needing a vocation for medicine have been eclipsed by an increasing emphasis on academic attainment. Little attention is paid to the personal characteristics of the potential doctor. And concern with the development of inter-personal skills in the training of doctors appears to be minimal.

There is, therefore, an interesting contrast between the doctors' and nurses' descriptions of the good nurse. It is a contrast which seems to be reflected in the attributes sought in the applicants to study nursing and medicine. Doctors-to-be need to have academic skills; nurses-to-be need to have suitable temperaments.

It is not surprising that both doctors and nurses emphasize the attributes which are valued within their own occupation. But it does mean that many doctors want nurses to be like doctors and, as will be seen below, many nurses similarly want doctors to be like nurses.

## THE GOOD DOCTOR

### The nurse's view

A 'good doctor' is good with patients. He takes time and care to explain to patients and their relatives what is going on. He doesn't stand at the end of the patient's bed making pronouncements. The good doctor interacts with the patient and is sensitive to the fears and lack of knowledge which patients have.*

He doesn't rush the patients; he's always got time to talk with them and he'll listen attentively to what they have to say. The good doctor has respect for, and listens to, the nurses. Indeed, he seeks nurses' advice, he consults them and is receptive to their opinions. For a few nurses, the good doctor must be competent and know what he is doing. But overall, in descriptions of the 'good doctor' the emphasis is upon his inter-personal skills rather than his skills as a medical practitioner. The good doctor seems also to be the good man and replicates the perfect hero of the pulp fiction so assiduously produced about doctors and nurses. The good man is caring and sensitive, yet strong, powerful and decisive.

'A nice attitude towards the patients. I mean you can tell he's thinking 'what a stupid woman this is' and yet he's absolutely super with her – nothing is too much trouble for them and that they'll sit and give them that little bit of extra time rather than just walk up and take a blood test. They'll walk up and sit and have a chat with her about her little cat or whatever – I think it's nice when they treat them as individuals and people, rather than just as a person sat in bed.' *Sister*

'I like it when they are thoughtful to the patients, nice to the patients, because a lot of them aren't. Again, they're not intentionally cruel, I don't mean that, but I think a lot of them forget to talk to the patients and one of the nicest things I ever remember when I was a student was an old lady was crying on the ward and one of the junior doctors

---

\* For an examination of the different expectations of various groups in the hospital as to the 'responsible' and 'irresponsible' doctor, refer to Loftus (1971).

went over with a box of tissues and sat down and said 'why are you crying' and was chatting away – well, they don't usually do things like that, they sort of run a mile if there's anything like that. That sort of thing impresses me. When they take time to talk to somebody.' *Staff Nurse*

'When they respect my opinion on a particular person's needs within health care; when they acknowledge my role on the ward as someone who can offer a particular service to the resident and yeah, not always directly to me, when they can acknowledge that the resident exists as a person. When they can sit down with that person and engage in a meaningful conversation with that person about their stay in hospital rather than to rely upon me to do it for them, rather than for me to interpret them to the patient, to the resident.' *Charge Nurse*

In many ways, the good doctor is a good father: thoughtful, kind and considerate. He has to do what a good father does: calms and reassures his children. 'Everything will be alright' and 'we're doing all we can', he says. Daddy knows what he's doing and he's doing all he can: we're safe in his hands.

## The doctor's view

For doctors, the 'good doctor' is a good clinician. Greatest respect is given to the clinical skills of a doctor. Any behaviour is tolerated if he's good with the knife or got a good brain on him. He'll be up to date with medical advances and all are assured that 'he will do a good job'. He can be recommended. He will also be decisive but approachable and willing to spend time with patients. Yet running a close second to the need for clinical skill is the importance of doctors' attitude to and relation with patients and their relatives. This emphasis on attitude was more often voiced by doctors in the most junior ranks: House Officers and Senior House Officers. It is, after all, in these grades that doctors have greatest contact with patients and relatives. At Consultant level, contact with patients is more formalized, with a tendency to be confined to the structured interactions during ward rounds and patient's visits to the out-patient department. Also, at Consultant level, there is relatively little opportunity for colleagues to scrutinize others' working practices, especially in relationships and demeanour towards patients. Clinical successes and failures are the things that are talked about in the dining room, not the manner in which Mr. So-and-so talks to his patients.

'First of all, they've got to be able to do the job that they're there for, be competent. They've got to be approachable – both from the nurses' point of view and from the patients' point of view . . . just do their job properly.' *Senior House Officer*

'I like conscientious young doctors who are keen to try out . . . who are confident enough to try out their own therapies on patients. I get annoyed when they are so widely wrong that they try the wrong thing out on patients, but I am very keen for good doctors to try out treatments because there is always more than one way of making a patient better.' *Consultant*

'Shows professional competence, knows his stuff, knows how to apply his stuff, and enthusiasm for the work and enthusiasm for the patient and sympathy for a patient, ideally without clouding judgment.' *Senior House Officer*

'Well, a good doctor should be somebody that knows their medicine, acts upon knowing their medicine and someone the patient feels they can freely talk to. And more so in terminal care because people have lots of fears and if you're unapproachable then no matter how many drugs you pump into them, it doesn't make any difference, so basically that you know what you're doing and that people can talk to you.' *Senior House Officer*

To some extent, the attributes valued in colleagues in the other occupation are the attributes valued within one's own occupation. This is especially true of nurses. The doctor with excellent clinical skills will be accorded respect, but it seems that the doctor with highly tuned inter-personal skills is likely to be given even more.

In seeking to find a reflection in the other group of the attributes valued within one's own group, the distinctive contributions which others have to offer may not be suffi-ciently recognized. If ideals were achieved and doctors, say, were to place even greater emphasis on their inter-personal skills, then nurses' special contribution as the 'people-centred', rather than disease-centred, occupation could be undermined.

## SUMMING UP

There is a contradiction within the accounts of the ideal types presented by nurses and doctors. Doctors say the good nurse is highly skilled and competent. They want nurses on whose judgement they can rely. Yet nurses frequently complain that their views are not listened to or sought by doctors. Nurses are treated as onlookers rather than participants in the treatment of patients. What these ideal types tell us is perhaps the failures of members of each occupational group to meet the expectations of others. Thus it seems, there is an implicit complaint that some doctors do not take sufficient time with, or fail to listen to, patients while some nurses do not exhibit, or are unwilling to develop, a reasonable level of skill in their work. It is hard to please everyone: there are few perfect partners.

# 8

# Listening and appreciating

One of the major reasons for the experience of inter-professional conflict is the perceived failure of doctors to seek, or to listen to, the opinions of nurses. The majority of doctors feel that they **do** listen to the opinions of nurses. Indeed, because of the greater knowledge which nurses have about the patients, doctors said they actively sought the opinions of nurses. Yet little more than a third of nurses felt that their opinions were listened to (Appendix Q). Comments about this aspect reveal many of the subtleties of the nurse-doctor interactions.

'They listen, yes, but nothing seems to get done and you are forever repeating yourself.' *Sister*

'Yes, as a Sister I feel they do. I know that my girls say "oh they won't listen to me, you will have to talk to them".' *Sister*

'Some doctors don't. I don't know why. Maybe its because they are too good to listen to what other people have got to say. I don't agree with that because I always find . . . well, it depends on the nurse. There are some that are very good. . . .' *Senior House Officer*

'Now certainly they ask my opinion. I mean they don't always take notice and I think you've always got to be careful that you don't overstep the mark because at the end of the day you know you are supposed to be carrying out the care that they prescribe.' *Staff Nurse*

'Believe it or not, the Consultants, I would say, are more

interested sometimes in what the nurses have got to say than the junior doctors.' *Staff Nurse*

'In intensive care, yeh, I would say they are listened to, and in theatre too, we rely by the nature of the job that we do, we rely quite a bit on the nursing staff on checking, or if we have to be called to the phone to monitor our patients.' *Registrar*

'All of the Consultants are fully prepared to listen to arguments on medical management put forward by nursing staff. I know in other units that this is a cause for disharmony . . . where nursing staff are considered to be there to do what they are told, and have no opinion on the management of patients. This is particularly so on long-term management on terminally ill patients as to whether, you know, one should continue with intensive management, or whether we should make them comfortable.' *Consultant*

'Wherever I have been the nurses have always been allowed, and I think that we have always listened to their comments, that's never been a problem.' *House Officer*

From nurses' and doctors' comments it is apparent that many factors influence the willingness to listen. Differences in the personality of the doctor, the grade of the doctor, the specialty are among the factors affecting whether doctors will seek, or listen to, the opinion of nurses. Consider the views of this Ward Sister and her Consultant:

'Sometimes you just . . . we realize that doctors are not listening to a word you are saying. That what you say does not count at all. They are the doctor and what they say is right and you know it is not right so if you have got the courage of your convictions and a large enough voice and you can stand up for yourself, you can fight it, but if you haven't and you're junior, you can forget it. Even if you are senior, you sometimes get browbeaten, so it doesn't always hold.' *Sister*

'The most important information you can get in hospital is from a nurse who says, "The patient's gone off a bit. . ." They are nursing the children, they are feeding them, they notice subtle changes before the doctors do and if they say baby so-and-so is not quite right today, we listen very carefully and it is ignored at the SHO's peril.' *Consultant*

There are obviously disparities in the accounts from the Sister and Consultant in this ward. Part of this disparity is accounted for by the different grades of doctor to which nurses have to relate. The Consultant may be keenly aware of the importance of listening to and seeking the opinions of nurses, and particularly Sisters. His Senior House Officer, however, may not accord importance to seeking nurses' opinions or even be aware of his Consultant's views on the matter. Again the length of time over which the nurse-doctor relationship has developed is an influencing factor. In the above ward, the Senior House Officers were often GP trainees having a brief experience of paediatrics as part of their training scheme. Not only are these SHOs' stay in paediatrics transitory, they are also not reliant on 'the reference' from the Consultant. The Consultant, therefore, wields less power and influence over the GP trainee in comparison with the junior doctor, whose hospital career centrally depends on the Consultant's reference.

The newly-qualified House Officer will listen most carefully to what nurses have to say. In fact, the new House Officer cannot survive without listening to nurses. However, in a few months' time, that House Officer will have gained in confidence, simultaneously downgrading the usefulness of any potential input from nurses. It is particularly irksome for nurses when a doctor who only last week dare not do anything without first asking a nurse, today refuses to listen to well-meant or useful advice. The failure to obtain information from the nursing staff will be noticed by this doctor's seniors. He is likely to be 'put in his place' in front of everyone: patient, colleagues and nurse. Beyond the most junior grades of doctors, there is great variability as regards willingness to listen to, or seek, the opinions of nurses.

## THE DOCTOR–NURSE GAME AGAIN

Often, in order to get information over, the 'doctor-nurse' game will be played. It can take place at any level, but is more likely to be played at junior doctor level. In this 'game' nurses have to disguise the fact that they are offering information, even advice, to doctors. At issue here is not a failure to listen, but a failure to give the nurse credit for her contribution.

'The nurses feel they have to phrase it in a certain way instead of just saying "why don't you use A", they'll say "the last time this patient was in they used drug A and they found the patient much better on that drug and I was wondering if possibly. . ." and they go through this whole rigmarole of taking three times as long to get to the same point because you know that if you suggest it. . .' *Sister*

'Oh yes, you have got to be very diplomatic, I mean you shouldn't be diagnosing or anything like that, a nurse is not trained for that. But you can pass opinion on things and depending on your surgeon, some of them would not be pleased and would do the opposite to what you suggest, depending on the way that you put it. You know if you suggest maybe a certain suture, they will use something completely different just to show that they are the surgeon and it's their decision what suture they will use.' *Theatre Sister*

### Offering opinions

Great care has to be taken by nurses in offering their opinions. They can so easily be taken 'the wrong way'. The prickliness of doctors to receiving information from others becomes apparent. They do not want to be seen as being in need of any assistance. They must not be seen as being influenced by others: their independence of thought and action must never come under question. The hedging around in the 'doctor-nurse' game ensures that nothing is said in a straightforward manner. The nurse's knowledge **is** wanted, but the nurse is not asked for it. Her competence is never revealed, and her opinion is not directly sought. She gains little from this game. The patient may gain quite a lot, or at least not lose anything by it. The doctor gains in three ways: he receives the coded information, he maintains his own dominant position and the superior knowledge of nurses can be disguised and overlooked. The rules of this game ensure that the nurse will never win: all the prizes go to the doctor.

Of course, some doctors do listen. Yet others are secure in

their own knowledge: there's little that any nurse can tell them: 'Well obviously I don't really see a need for it, I mean I think that it is my job to ask really' (*Consultant*). There are some doctors who do not recognize at all their need of nurses' input. These doctors will have their competence questioned by nurses: an exquisite agony for the conceited junior doctor. Such a doctor will in turn be accused of not having the patient's interests at heart. Indeed such a doctor is putting protection of his own ego before his patients. Bad doctors do not listen and they sometimes cannot listen because of the status of the person who has the information to give. 'They will not listen to you because you are only a nurse. Your opinion doesn't count because you a nurse' (*Staff Nurse*). Such doctors maintain their own professional dignity at the expense of nurses, and even more so at the expense of patients.

The doctors will say that some nurses are not worth listening to, they make stupid or irrelevant suggestions and don't understand the problems involved. And the useful information offered by nurses will be thrown out with the useless. There are many reasons why the opinions of nurses are not sought. The different emphases in training, the different types of skills and the different priorities regarding health care in medicine and nursing mean that information offered is often perceived to be useless or irrelevant. Nurses are felt to lack appreciation of the difficulties doctors face in the treatment and management of patients.

## Accepting opinions

Whether or not a nurse's opinion is listened to depends in large measure on her experience. The recently-qualified Staff Nurse is likely to find that any opinions or suggestions she proffers will not be attended to. On the other hand, the Ward Sister with many years' experience of the specialty and of working with the same Consultant(s) will find that she is listened to closely.

Thus, whether nurses are new to their post, whether their opinion or views are to be trusted, whether they offer the information the 'right way', whether they are forceful in offering their opinions are some of the variables affecting the extent to which nurses are listened to.

Teaching hospital nurses, especially those in London, were felt to be more assertive and less acquiescent to doctors than their colleagues in non-teaching hospitals. This may be related to the more 'aggressive' treatment pursued in teaching hospitals and the presence of more assertive nurses with a higher sense of self-esteem. Scottish nurses gave the strong impression of being more deferential and acquiescent to members of the medical profession. Some nurses are more obviously supportive of a 'medical' view of the patient. As Owens and Glennerster (1990, p.39) remind us, 'It is important to remember that the nurse has always worked closely with the doctors, and has, therefore, become gradually more orientated to the medical model of care.' A distinct nursing view of the world is still in the process of formation, and many rank and file nurses seem to be 'doctors' nurses' rather than 'nurses' nurses'. These 'doctors' nurses' are unlikely to speak out or to feel the need to speak out about doctors' decisions. The doctor is not to be questioned. That many nurses should subscribe to a 'medical model' of care is not surprising. It is, after all, within the hospital that the great majority of nurses find employment. The hospital is tailor-made for the medical profession: it is an environment in which the preferences of the medical profession dominate. Nurses, initially barely tolerated by doctors, have traditionally been grateful to doctors for their inclusion in the hospital world. (The gains which Florence Nightingale was able to make, in establishing nursing alongside the medical profession, were accomplished at a cost, one which is still being paid.) There was a reflected glory for nurses in their association with the medical profession. For some nurses, this reflected glory remains a welcome reality and for them doctors can do little wrong. This type of nurse has been identified by Katz (1969, p.68) as a 'traditionalizer' who 'takes an uncritical stance with regard to knowledge and existing practices in the hospital: she is a guardian, not a harnesser; she mainly guards the traditions of the hospital and the physicians.' The idea that a doctor-nurse game is being played is often misleading. Indeed, in many instances it seems to be wishful thinking. The games that have been found in accident and emergency departments (Hughes, 1988a,b) are much less in evidence in care of the elderly wards. Indeed, nurses often do not speak up and do not offer information which is potentially useful in making a decision on the management of a patient. The British Medical Association (1981, p.43) is aware of the need for nurses to voice their opinions: 'In cases in which nurses' continuous contact with the patient has given them a different insight into the patient's medical needs, they are under a moral obligation to communicate this to the doctor in charge of the case.'

Nurses' silence condemns them. They may mutter to junior doctors about some particular decision, yet will not themselves speak out and say clearly what they think (Roberts, 1983; Smith, 1987a). They allow themselves to be overawed and silenced. And by their silence, nurses do not help the patient or the relatives. Nurses' silence simply gives additional support to medical power (Gardner and McCoppin, 1986) and restricts patients' power. To a substantial extent, the stance taken by the Ward Sister in encouraging nurses to question doctors will determine the willingness of nurses to voice their opinions. Revans (1962, p.125) also has noted the negative influence of Sisters with regard to student nurses asking doctors questions. Quite a few nurses and doctors mentioned this reluctance of some nurses to voice their opinion. Nurses, it seems, can be their own worst enemy. While Blanche (1988, p.157) feels that nursing students would speak out if it was 'a matter of life and death', it appears that a few of the qualified nurses interviewed would not.

It is easy to blame nurses for their quiescence. Some nurses have been outspoken and vociferous, as they know to their own cost. But nurses are only part of the equation. The other part is the way in which nurses can be, and are, humiliated publicly by some doctors. Shouted at in front of patients and relatives, ridiculed as newly-qualified nurses for their lack of knowledge of some medical term, silenced by the glare of an autocratic doctor, it is not surprising if there is a reluctance to speak out. Some doctors take a delight in finding fault with nurses and in so doing, asserting their own superiority and power. When a 'dressing-down' is given in front of a patient, nurses will seldom answer back. They know the rules that the doctor must not be contradicted in front of the patient. The doctor may be spoken to later, but it cannot remove the earlier embarrassment or humiliation of the nurse. There is no doubt that senior doctors enjoy the luxury of being able to express their anger in their relationships with nurses and junior doctors:

'Just as a senior person enjoying the privilege of being able to be ill tempered at times when other people are bound to suppress it. . .' *Consultant*

Whether or not senior doctors capitalize on their ability to display their irritation or anger depends greatly on their own personal style of working, and to some extent, on the specialty in which they work.

## THE 'GREAT-I-AM'

The majority of doctors and nurses felt that a substantial number of doctors suffer from the affliction of the 'Great-I-Am' (Appendix R). This condition manifests itself in a variety of ways and with differing degrees of success according to the grade of the doctor. While nearly half the doctors thought that this problem was confined to junior doctors, only a third of nurses thought this was the case. Only a small number of nurses said there was no problem with this projection of 'greatness' among medical staff, and almost all of them worked in Scotland.

This display of superiority is called many things. There is the 'white-coat-itis' of the newly-qualified doctor, euphoric at their own success in getting through medical school and their future career prospects. They clearly feel themselves to be superior to nursing staff and make it quite apparent. Although nurses will 'deal with' an arrogant junior doctor, it may make little difference in the long run. 'Great' doctors seem to be born, not made, and there is little chance of changing some of them. If there are no confident and experienced nurses to tell them off, these juniors will continue to use their bullying tactics as they progress up the hospital career ladder. As medical students they will have been told almost daily how they are the intellectual elite, the top 1% in the country, and when they finally qualify they want others to acknowledge their elevated position and that they are in fact God's gift to medicine. It is in their attitude towards nurses that they may come unstuck. (It is worth noting that not one person talked about doctor's demeanour towards patients in this context.) If junior doctors refuse to listen, won't take advice or aren't at all helpful, they may find they are 'dropped in it' on the ward round. It can be a particularly painful experience.

'It can stop the ward, everything goes silent and everybody else listens to what is going on, patients and staff alike. . . . the best scene that I ever saw was down in [X]. . . a House Officer who had been sort of particularly obstructive towards the nursing staff was dropped in it by the Sister, and promptly hauled over the coals by one of the worst . . . well a Consultant who has the best choice of language I have ever heard, in a public place. I mean it was a male House Officer and he was reduced to tears, and he certainly changed his attitude towards the nursing staff after that, they never had any problems with him again.' *Senior House Officer*

### Temper and arrogance

At more senior levels, the inflated status of some doctors manifests itself not only in general demeanour, but also in displays of temper. There is a clear division within the ranks of Consultants between those who adopt a 'reasonable' demeanour and those who don't. The 'prima donna' performance in the operating theatre so well portrayed by Sir Launcelot Spratt in the *Doctor-in-the-House* films, all too readily reflects the behaviour of some Consultants. As mentioned earlier, Consultants do not have to contain their feelings. The tensions inherent in working at a senior level, making difficult and life-depending decisions are reason enough for some displays of emotion. At the same time, however, Consultants can be unnecessarily impatient, tyrannical, dictatorial, rude and dismissive of others. They can, in other words, misuse their position of power and authority. Why should some Consultants do this? There are number of influences at work here.

Firstly, nurses themselves foster Consultant's superiority in that nurses kowtow to these Consultants' expectation of a special dispensation in the way they behave. This expectation is, in large part, understandable. Consultants undertake highly specialized work in relative isolation from others. There is no one in a position to question Consultants' knowledge or practice. They easily become highly eccentric if they want to because there isn't a great deal of pressure that can be exerted upon them to change their behaviour if it becomes odd. Being arrogant can function as a defence mechanism. Doctors who begin to question their own decisions would find life almost intolerable. The awful possibility that wrong decisions have been made presents an onerous burden. That possibility is faced in isolation with little chance of open discussion of doubt with colleagues in other specialties. It is little wonder, therefore, that so many doctors need to ease their burden with alcohol and mental breakdowns. Human beings are not designed to play God, a role in which patients and some nurses are only too keen to place Consultants. It is a particularly cruel irony that doctors are blamed for playing God when that is the role assigned to them by others. The abdication of responsibility by patients (and some nurses) means that someone else has to take that responsibility.

The few Registrars and Senior Registrars, who strut and swagger as though Lord-of-the-Manor, are preparing themselves for a future exalted position as Consultant. Medicine is highly competitive and the top places go to the best. In order to convince yourself and others that you are deserving of a top place you behave like those at the top. Some Registrars wait until they become Consultants before they start behaving like one. Today's Consultants act as role models for their juniors, a few of whom will become the Consultants of the future. The style affected by Consultants is not always attractive, at least to nursing staff (or patients!). For example, in the professorial units in teaching hospitals, the postures adopted by the senior Consultants have been described as producing a 'nightmarish' atmosphere.

To accompany such a grandiose view of oneself, others necessarily have to be relegated to inferior positions. Thus, nurses can be viewed as second class citizens and certainly not to be asked their opinions regarding the management of patient care. In turn the posture adopted by Consultants explains some of the reluctance of nurses to offer their opinions.

The case must not be overstated. The majority of Consultants are quite reasonable in their behaviour. Not for them the throwing about of case notes, the dramatic outburst or the impatient drumming of fingers as they wait for a nurse to accompany them on their ward round. These Consultants make no grand entrances on to the ward, they are quiet and respectful of the perspectives of others. Even for these Consultants, some nurses are silent and will not offer their opinions. An unwillingness to assert themselves, carefully engendered in nurse training is compounded by nurses' refusal to see themselves as partners in the delivery of health care.

## HOW DOCTORS AND NURSES SEE EACH OTHER

### Nurses' views of doctors

A small number of doctors and nurses (29 and 24 respectively) were asked how they felt nurses in general saw doctors. The aim was to uncover some of the prejudices and aspirations of respondents that they might not wish to give in response to a direct and more personal question. Most noticeable in the answers was the perception that nurses viewed the medical profession with awe or subservience. Although a few mentioned the respect in which nurses held the medical profession, others felt some nurses are antagonistic to doctors.

### Doctors' views of nurses

Thirty-seven doctors and 71 nurses were asked how they felt nurses generally were seen by doctors. Again, it was associations with subservience and handmaids that were most often mentioned. Nurses certainly were not seen as equals by these doctors. A few viewed nurses with respect and only a small number viewed nurses with antagonism.

These describing words of 'subservience', 'antagonism' and 'respect' are the ones used by doctors and nurses. They reflect the reality of the relationship between nurses and doctors. Nurses were keenly aware of their subordinate relationship to doctors. However, it was nurses who were identified (by nurses) as being to blame for their own subordination. Doctors were not identified as being responsible in any way for the subservience of nurses.

'They [nurses] are absolutely mummified by this subservientness. They don't see it like that, but I do, I just don't understand how you can work in an area like this and still just be a bum washer, I just can't understand it.' *Staff Nurse, trained in Australia*

'As a generalization I think they just see them as a sort of skivvy to do the sort of fetch and carry things. . .' *Senior House Officer*

There is a critical element missing from many of these general descriptions of the other occupation. Those who comment about the inferiority of nurses don't go on to mention the superiority of doctors. The power of the medical profession is disguised by placing emphasis on the response of nurses to that power. In this way nurses can be seen as their own worst enemy and the dynamics of power and status can be ignored.

## HOW THEY OUGHT TO BEHAVE

There is no doubt whatsoever, that most nurses want doctors to treat them with respect and to be seen as equals and colleagues. Doctors should be courteous, listen to what nurses have to say and appreciate their knowledge. Doctors, on the other hand, stress the importance of respect but they lay less emphasis on treating nurses as equals and colleagues.

'Well, as fellow professionals, and as human beings as well, I mean everyone has got feelings, there is no point in bawling out a nurse because she has forgotten to do the ECG that you asked her to do or whatever, I mean you just say 'well perhaps you could do it now'. There's no point in getting over angry with people, you should treat them with the respect that you expect to be treated yourself.' *Senior House Officer*

'I think that they [doctors] should appreciate the work that they are doing, and in turn they should be pleasant as well and make their nurses' life a lot easier, treat them with respect as well. But it is difficult believe me.' *House Officer*

'You have to let them know who's boss.' *Registrar*

'I think as part of a team. I mean if you try to say you are the boss I don't think that helps . . . they are just as important as you, because, I mean, in a way they are.' *Female Registrar*

'I think first of all you shouldn't be rude to nurses. I think you are asking for trouble if you do that. They deserve respect. A lot of them have been psychiatric nurses for a long, long time. They have got a lot more experience of psychiatry than I have I am sure. I have only been doing it for four months. That's it really.' *Senior House Officer*

'I think tolerance and give-and-take on both sides, I don't think that the nurses should kowtow to everything we say, and I don't think that we should bend over backwards for everything that they say, I think it has got to be on both sides.' *Registrar*

'I certainly feel for myself that if you want to look after your patients in the best possible way you've got to make the nurse feel comfortable about communicating with you and if she has you on a pedestal she won't.' *Senior House Officer*

It was apparent that some younger doctors paid only lip-service to treating nursing staff as colleagues. Their view of nurses was essentially negative. Thus doctors were not to be rude, not to bawl at nurses, not to explicitly say that the doctor is boss. The underlying message is: contain your anger and impatience when dealing with these inferior beings.

'I don't think a lot of nurses appreciate the fact that a lot of the doctor's actions are not through bloody-mindedness, because they don't know any different, that's how they have been trained. I think a bit more tolerance and respect, because as I said before you will not receive respect if you never give it.' *Staff Nurse*

'Well I think they should be friendly towards me, not try and boss me about and treat me like servants. . .' *Male Staff Nurse*

'As an equal I think, as somebody that you are working with, not somebody who is working for you.' *Sister*

'I think they ought to treat us just as equals really and realize that the job we do is just as important as theirs and without each other the patient can't benefit really.' *Sister*

The need for nurses not to treat **themselves** as subservient was repeated frequently. It was evident from many comments that nurses do not see themselves as equals of doctors. This finding is not new (Mackay, 1989, p.181) but is surprising that it still emerges strongly regarding registered nurses as distinct from enrolled and student nurses. The nurses' requests for respect and courtesy from medical colleagues were not meant to refute the inequality of doctors and nurses.

'I think nurses should still be respectful to doctors, but I don't think doctors should be treated like tin gods.. Because after all, we're here to give a service to the patient.' *Sister*

'We need to determine what our roles are, how we see each other and realize that you should respect each other without having to be the Yes Sir, No Sir, bit – that's grovelling. You have got to be able to respect each other and respect each other's point of view.' *Staff Nurse*

'I like someone who is aggressive back, I like somebody who will treat me as an equal and doesn't treat me as someone on a pedestal, I mean the fact that I am a Senior Registrar doesn't mean I am any different from . . . we are all in here together, it just happens that I have got a bit more responsibility than them.' *Senior Registrar*

'They [nurses] should treat them the same really – with respect again and not be wary of them. If there was something drastically wrong they could feel that they could put it forward.' *Sister*

## THE DIFFERENCES IN WHAT THEY DO

The way in which doctors and nurses describe the difference in their work clearly illustrates the inequality in their relationship (Mackay, 1992a). For most nurses and doctors, it seems that nurses do what doctors tell them to; that the doctor directs, controls and decides on patient care. Nurses carry out doctors' orders. Nurses undertake the practical and basic care of patients. 'Doctors', in the words of one surgical House Officer, 'do the brainwork, while nurses do the legwork'. However, for a few, nurses were elevated to a role of acting as the eyes and ears of doctors in their absence. Working together, as a team, was seldom mentioned.

The difference between what nurses and doctors are seen to do is also reflected in the focus of their 'gaze' (Foucault, 1973). Nurses are identified as being concerned with the 'whole' patient, with the psychological, emotional and social aspects of patient care. Doctors, on the other hand, are seen as being primarily concerned with the clinical aspects of patient care. Perhaps not surprisingly, it was nurses who mentioned a role for the nurse in the diagnosis and assessment of patients.

### Diagnostic roles

Psychiatry is the specialty in which the nurse's diagnostic role was most often mentioned. The more intimate and intensive contact that psychiatric nurses have with patients ensures that they are particularly well placed to evaluate changes in the patients' emotions and state of mind. It is not simply that psychiatric nurses act as doctors' 'eyes and ears', they have to act, indeed they are trained to act, in the absence of doctors. This freedom is also enjoyed within highly specialized units such as Intensive Therapy, Coronary Care, Accident and Emergency.

To some extent all nurses must undertake some patient assessment. It is nursing staff who are likely to notice any changes in patient colour, temperature or pulse. Decisions to call a doctor have to be made and to that extent, nurses themselves evaluate the patient's condition. Failure to take action is potentially extremely serious. There is, in this way, some overlap between the roles of nurse and doctor. Their respective roles can be blurred: there is a 'grey' area of practice which is infrequently mentioned by both doctors and nurses.

The quality of the doctor–nurse relationship matters tremendously. Routine decisions are relatively easy and there will be mutually accepted ways of proceeding in such cases. Some decisions are anything but routine and they need a cool head. There is great need for objectivity in such decisions. Personal, subjective feelings must be discounted. Emotion clouds the intellect, and emotion offers a particular threat to an intellect which prides itself on objective and rational 'scientific' knowledge. However, it is not always possible to view patients objectively, especially when personal knowledge of the patient has been gained. Greater contact with, and a deeper knowledge of, a patient can complicate decision-making. This may be why a contribution from nurses to patient management decisions is not sought. Nurses, through their greater closeness with patients are likely to be swayed by their personal feelings.

Doctors have to block highly emotional information, it is one of their defence mechanisms (Young, 1981, p.151). This 'blocking' is reasonable. Subjective, emotional and 'feeling' information cannot make medical decision-making easier. It is not 'scientific', it is not 'rigorous' and it can introduce irrelevant considerations. Doctors want objective knowledge. Yet, doctors do rely on such intuitive judgements from nurses, particularly when nurses 'know' there is something wrong with a patient which is not revealed by any of the observations or monitoring being conducted. Thus, some doctors know to respond quickly to the 'feelings' of some nurses. The 'uncanny' knowledge is, and can be, valuable. These 'hunches' are in fact an integral part of the **art** of nursing (Uprichard, 1971, p.230).

This type of knowledge is 'knowledge in action' (Benner, 1984; Schon, 1987), learned through experience and not through the lecture or seminar. It is knowledge which is hard to describe. Like riding a bike, the 'feel' of a diseased organ or the 'look' of a patient defies description. There is little recognition of such knowledge in nurses' and doctors' definitions of the differences between what they do. The emphasis is on the observable and the definable. (In accounts of the 'good nurse' however, the need to be able to trust a nurse's judgement was often mentioned. This judgement is 'the hunch', the feeling that something, unobserved and unobservable is 'wrong'.)

In a similar way, the level of knowledge that a doctor or nurse possesses is not always apparent: it is knowledge which can only be observed or appreciated 'in action'. It is obviously important to individuals to have these competencies and skills recognized. The patients have their own ideas as to how to differentiate between the highly competent doctor from the less competent. Nurses also can do that. And doctors can similarly differentiate between the competent and less competent nurse. Colleagues' perceptions of competence are extremely important.

## BEING APPRECIATED

The nurses and doctors interviewed would very much like to have their workload and their stresses appreciated by their colleagues. There were many heartfelt cries from junior doctors about nurses' lack of recognition about the demands of their job.

Nurses feel they appreciate doctors' workload (Appendix S). However, only a minority of doctors feel that their workload is appreciated (Appendix T). Some nurses said they knew how tired the doctors became, how impossible the hours were and how hard the junior doctors worked. It was quite clear, however, that a substantial number of nurses did not appreciate the special strains inherent in junior doctors' work. These nurses seemed uninterested and unconcerned about the demands placed on junior doctors. There was a job to be done and the House Officer had to do it.

Doctors were more confident that *they* appreciated nurses' work and indeed, over half the nurses agreed that doctors did appreciate the stresses and strains involved in their work.

Doctors felt that nurses' lack of understanding was most noticeable regarding junior doctors' hours and the intolerable strain associated with being on call. Doctors seemed keen to defend themselves against charges of being lazy. The hassling and constant reminding to which some doctors were subjected by nurses was obviously felt to contain an implicit message that doctors weren't doing anything. Yet very few nurses mentioned lazy doctors, it wasn't an issue for them. What was an issue for nurses was that doctors couldn't be found when they were wanted: they were never there, or they didn't answer their bleep. Slightly double-edged comments made about colleagues' workload illustrated the tension between wanting appreciation, yet not being prepared to give it oneself.

'I appreciate they [doctors] do a lot of hours, especially on call at weekends and if you are ringing up at 3 o'clock in the early hours of Sunday morning, it's not a good time, if they have been on call since Friday. But, at the end of the day, they are still there to do a job of work and if I have got a problem at that time I expect – but then again a lot of nursing staff will ring them up for really trivial things at inappropriate times. So it goes both ways. They can be quite annoyed with the nursing staff and rightly so at times.' *Staff Nurse*

'The Registrar is very busy because she flits between here and [another hospital] and various domiciliary visits, so it comes back down to the House Officer, who if they are really conscientious can get lumbered with an awful lot of things to deal with in any one day. And then they are at the beck and call of the bleeper. And I would say that they are under extreme pressure, and there is this on-call business going all over the weekend. I actually have quite a lot of sympathy for House Officers, much as they do do silly things sometimes, I wouldn't have their job.' *Staff Nurse*

'The thing that really annoys me sometimes about nurses is they don't appreciate the number of hours we do at all, and very often their attitude is unpleasant . . . the problems I think arise because you have to be on so many wards at one time, and if a nurse phones you up and says, 'can you do this, can you come and see this patient?', and you say, 'well I can't I've more important things to do', then their attitude is often, it often becomes aggressive, and you know, they want you immediately, and you have to explain you're too busy.' *Senior House Officer*

'I think some [doctors] do and some don't. People who don't are those who are still caught up in their own work and are over-run with thinking about this and that and they are just trying to get by the day and they don't really have much energy for anyone but themselves.' *Senior House Officer*

Wanting other people to know how busy you are, what its like doing your job cannot be dismissed as self-indulgent or self-pitying. If we are not appreciated through the work we do, we experience a lack of motivation. Considerable appreciation for the work of nurses and doctors can, and does, come from patients. However, patients are temporary, they move through the hospital at ever greater speed. Recovery takes place in the hospital, but recuperation increasingly takes place at home. Long gone are the days when the patients were in a condition to help nursing staff with their daily chores. There are few long-stay patients now. And there are less likely to be those ward 'worthies' and 'characters' who fully and warmly appreciate the work and demands placed on junior doctors and on nurses. The boxes of chocolates are still to be found at the nurses' station: patients are still appreciative, but have less opportunity to express it. This rapid throughput of patients and the accompanying intensification of work means that the opinions of colleagues become increasingly important. If colleagues do not appreciate your workload, then they are likely to make ever-greater demands of you. For example, there is a great deal of work involved for nurses in carrying out half-hourly observations on patients. If a doctor does not appreciate how much additional work each request for this causes, then his recommendations for such monitoring of patients may well be met with resentment and anger. The doctor will find that he is being bleeped about trifling matters. He will become impatient and angry with the nurses who don't seem to appreciate just how busy he is and how many demands there are on his time. If the nurse does not realize how awful it is to be wakened about trivial matters in the middle of the night, she will soon find that her credibility as a nurse declines rapidly. Whatever requests she makes will be dealt with irritating slowness. And the doctor will find he continues to be wakened about matters which an appreciative nurse could easily leave until morning.

### Failure to appreciate

There is, therefore, a considerable price to be paid for a lack of appreciation of the workload and demands being placed on colleagues. Not only will people try to 'get their own back' on those who are seen to have wronged them, but everyone will experience greater stress in their own working lives. There will be inter-personal tensions and a growing inability to work cooperatively with colleagues. Attitudes to the other group as

a whole will also suffer. No matter how good, how appreciative, how thoughtful the new doctor or the new nurse is, it will
not do them any good. They will be seen negatively and
classed with their unappreciative predecessors. Awkward and
unhelpful inter-professional relations can easily be translated
into a lack of respect for the other and the work they do. It
would be surprising if patient care was unaffected by these
tensions. Tasks performed for the patient which were re-
quested by 'that' doctor may be done with ill-grace. Relatives
to whom 'that' nurse has asked the doctor to speak may be
dealt with cursorily or with impatience. An inevitable
downward spiral soon sets in motion.

The failure to appreciate the stresses and work of colleagues
in part stemmed from generalized perceptions of the other
occupation. Nurses were seen as handmaidens, even servants,
of the medical profession. From this it followed that all that
nurses did was to tidy, clean and wipe bottoms. The
association of nurses with 'dirty work' and the corresponding
need to distance themselves from such low-status work meant
that quite a few junior doctors were particularly dismissive of
nurses and their work. Exceedingly negative views of nurses
were encountered, it seems, in medical school and some young
doctors were unwilling or unable to revise those views
(Webster, 1985).

'When you are on the big ward and that they just don't see
that you've got any brains or you're just there to clean the
patients, bedbath them, clean them up when they've made a
mess and feed them. They probably don't realize that you're
probably the one that looks at the results and thinks "oh, this
isn't quite right, I'll just ring them up to do this". They don't
realize that side of it.' *Sister*

'In medical school the view is that they are there to fetch and
carry and shovelling shit and sputums, sort of thing.' *Senior
House Officer*

'Some people come in thinking they can treat their
colleagues and nursing staff you know as muck, if you take
that, some will try and walk all over you.' *Staff Nurse*

'I don't think they see them [nurses], I don't even think if
they see them as professionals sometimes, I don't know. I

don't think that they think they are as important as medical staff.' *Sister*

As students, it seems that nurses view doctors, all doctors, with awe and as someone to be looked up to but not to speak to. Once qualified and having found her feet, the nurse may revise and wish to establish a different relationship with members of the medical profession. Yet it seems that many nurses are not able to reappraise their view of doctors who remain on a pedestal, unapproachable and superior. Such nurses are unable to leave behind the attitudes which were so regularly reinforced as students.

'Some of them tend to be quite subservient and look up to you because you're a doctor, but I don't really like that. I think they should talk to you on the same level.' *House Officer*

'The student nurses, a lot of them sort of hold you in awe, and if you talk to them they just sort of look at you sort of "gosh it's a doctor" kind of thing.' *Senior House Officer*

'Because we haven't got the same knowledge and understanding that doesn't mean that we are any less of a person, and it's difficult to say what I mean. I think they do treat you as if you're inferior to them, and I think that they really think that you are, and we **are** in knowledge and understanding, but I think, if they took the time to explain to us exactly why they were doing things then we wouldn't appear so silly to them.' *Staff Nurse*

'In the wards, when the Consultants would come in for their ward rounds and that would maybe be all that you saw of them. And you would bow down to them as if they were somebody important.' *Staff Nurse, ITU*

### Overcoming the problem

The inability to confront received opinions gained in training results in a blindness to the work of the other. The stereotypes are blinkers which critically affect working relationships and working practices. If you cannot appreciate the fallibility and lack of confidence of the junior doctor, you may be asking too much of him, pushing him into a omnipotent role that he doesn't want to fill. If you cannot appreciate the importance of the nurse as the doctor's observer on the wards, then you may be asking too little of her, pushing her into a restrictive role and denying her any independence of action.

It is as junior doctors and nurses that the negative views of colleagues must be addressed. Because of the amount of contact, poor views of colleagues and a lack of mutual appreciation make working lives miserable. And if negative views are not addressed as juniors, when a substantial amount of contact takes place, they are unlikely to be addressed when the contact is reduced. Moving up the career ladder takes both away from the patient and from members of the other occupation. Negative views can then become fixed for the rest of their careers. The underlying plea from so many junior doctors and nurses was, 'If only they could understand what it is like to have this job.' There is no doubt that some nurses and some doctors do not know, and some do not *want* to know about the workload of their nursing or medical colleagues.

It was clear that others were in a position to fully appreciate the demands and tensions involved in their colleagues' work. Their particular understanding of doctors or nurses work is gained from three different sources.

First, there is the knowledge gained from partners and friends who work in the other occupation. Doctors who are married to nurses are likely to be made aware of the grouses and groans about doctors. Nurses who have to put up with their fiancé's on-call hours and vitriolic comments about nurses who refuse to use their initiative, are likely to think twice about bleeping a doctor. Twenty of the fifty doctors who were asked about their spouse's/partner's occupation said that they were nurses (a further 11 doctors' partners were doctors). Five of the 47 nurses asked this question were married to doctors. It seems from this that considerable numbers of doctors and nurses will have heard the views of their colleagues at first-hand!

Secondly, for both doctors and nurses, a particular appreciation is gained when they themselves are patients. The keenly-awaited drink that is put just out of reach of the immobilized orthopaedic patient will be long remembered. Particularly thoughtful accounts of his experiences as a patient have been made by Sacks (1986, p.132) who argues the need for a doctor to be 'a patient among patients.' The experience of being a patient can obviously be influential. Four of the doctors and eight nurses took up their careers due to their own or a family member's illness. Some medical students are given experience as a patient for one day. A professor in a London teaching hospital was reputed to make all his students spend one whole day in a wheelchair, which they're not allowed to leave to go to the toilet or do anything without first requesting someone to come. There's nothing like first-hand experience to consolidate learning.

Thirdly, working in hospitals as a porter or nursing auxiliary can give medical students invaluable insight into what really happens in the ward. The routines, the incessant and never-ending demands made on nurses, the way in which doctors comport themselves, are revealed and understood (Richards, 1983). Most medical students are now given some experience of working at ward level on the 'nursing' side. (The benefits of working on the nursing side have been extolled by many commentators, such as Bowers, 1970, and Atkinson, 1976.) The experience they are given is seldom extensive, it ranges from a couple of weeks to one day where they 'get the feel of' a particular ward. Some doctors obviously gain a substantial amount of understanding through their ward experience. Others find it 'a laugh', while some of their fellow students will avoid it altogether. As in everything, those medical students who are potentially receptive towards the experience will gain most from it. Those who think such experience is a waste of time, learn nothing. That some medical students are so disdainful of the activities of nurses and the experiences of patients, should surely be a cause for concern among senior members of the medical profession. Should these students have been allowed to embark on a medical career?

While nearly two thirds of the nurses felt it would be a good idea for medical students to spend some time working on the 'nursing side', only one third of doctors agreed (Appendix U). A smaller number of doctors and nurses were also asked what they felt about nurses 'shadowing' a junior doctor for a few days to see what it was like being on call and having a bleep. There was a surprising amount of enthusiasm for the idea from both nurses and doctors with around two thirds in favour of it (Appendix V).

'I think that would be quite an eye-opener for us just to see what it was like. They are up (out of bed/awake). Especially the housemen, they tend to get the brunt of it. When I did B block, you sort of have got this poor houseman and they have been qualified one or two months and they are suddenly expected, they are on their tod, and especially if they haven't got an understanding Registrar, or SHO, and they are in at the deep end.' *Staff Nurse*

'I think it would give them a little bit of insight . . . a lot of the junior staff they don't really realize the hassles of having to change somebody's bed every hour of the day, clear up all the soiled linen, . . . 'shovelling shit' they call it, it must be horrific for the girls to do it so many times in the day and still keep a smile on their face. So there are things that both sides can learn from, seeing what happens on the shop floor.' *Senior Registrar*

'My first job after qualifying I worked in Special Suite X-Ray because I was waiting for this Surgical post to come up and I had a bleep. I was on-call one weekend in three for road traffic accidents and things like that, so I understood the whole world of carrying a bleep and being woken up in the night and one weekend I will never forget. I was called in 18 times! So I feel I have got a little bit more insight into what it means when you are bleeped for really stupid things.' *Staff Nurse*

'I think that it [would] introduce them to a more realistic approach to patient care. I think wiping bottoms, and the intimate care is something that they have to appreciate is important to patients, and it is something that brings them closer to patients, and probably also closer to an understanding of how nurses perceive patients.' *Senior Registrar*

'On some wards they will be over-used and the person in charge may vent their frustrations that they've developed from doctors and vented it on the poor medical student who has come up to the ward.' *Staff Nurse*

'Oh, that would be a good idea for a number of reasons. It is my idea of what a mill-owner would do with his son, he would send him down to start sweeping a broom and work from the shopfloor up, just to get an idea. I worked as a hospital porter for some time which I found a really valuable experience.' *Consultant*

Even if medical and nursing education were to wholeheartedly embrace the idea of 'seeing the world as the other sees it', this could not overcome the attitudes that are already entrenched within the system. It is senior doctors and senior nurses who are most likely to act as role models in the behaviour that is adopted by the newly-qualified doctors and nurses. It is the practices and attitudes displayed by those who hold the keys to career and promotion which are influential in changing behaviour.

In focusing on the divergent perspectives of nurses and doctors it is easy to overlook the extent to which they share a common experience in the work they do. From many comments it was apparent that there is a great deal in which doctors and nurses do share. Both share in their experience of working in that hospital. To both, the hospital is where they work and where they may feel at ease. They share their knowledge and experience of working for the NHS: that slow-moving and convoluted bureaucracy which they love to hate. They have a common understanding of the world of intrigue and gossip that is the hospital. They share a knowledge of how the hospital works, what is done to patients, and what each medical condition entails. They have a shared understanding of why they are there. They face similar pressures with the trauma of the dying patient and similar rewards in the joys of recovery. They share conversations about their daily activities from which outsiders are necessarily excluded. They share a taste for 'gallows humour' which helps them cope with the bad road traffic accident and the ghastliness of what they have to witness.

'It's us against the world: the people involved in health care – that's nurses and doctors and not others. It is a privilege to see people as patients. We see them when they are naked. We learn a lot about them. It is a privilege and we have a special role and we do see something special together.' *Consultant*

Although they may complain about the lack of understanding and appreciation among their nursing and medical colleagues, there is no one who can better understand their working life than these same colleagues. There are no others more fitted to support and encourage them than their working partners. Every attempt must be made to do so.

# 9

# Abandoning gender

Much has been made of the importance of gender in defining the roles and status of nurses and doctors. Nurses are subordinate to doctors because they are women. And doctors are superior because they are men. It all seems so simple. But it doesn't explain the dynamics of the doctor-nurse relationship for male nurses and female doctors.

Nursing is associated with women. Medicine is associated with men. Male nurses and female doctors are people who are, to some extent, out of place. Their gender will tend to be mentioned in any casual conversations about them. Nurses ought to be women and doctors ought to be men.

Although in the past, women have had to struggle to get into medicine (Bell, 1953), women now account for nearly half of the medical students and have managed to establish themselves in reasonable numbers in some hospital specialties. However, women continue to struggle to get into particular bastions of male power in specialties such as surgery and obstetrics and gynaecology (Allen, 1988; Parkhouse, 1991). Even special talents with which women have so long been associated, like manual dexterity, so desirable in some surgical specialties, have not been sufficient to counter the contamination of their gender (Young, 1981).

## MALES IN NURSING

Men account for around 10% of nurses (a proportion which has not risen noticeably in recent years). Traditionally, men were found in psychiatric nursing which has its own history and tradition (Brown and Stones, 1973). The restraining and custodial role of the care given to mental patients has ensured men a place because of their physical strengths. There is a strong connection between the work of prison officers and the early attendants in psychiatric hospitals.

Male nurses have had a particular struggle in gaining access to general nursing. There seem to be few male nurses in paediatrics or in obstetrics and gynaecology. Their gender ensures their exclusion: sometimes on the grounds of delicacy, at other times to protect the monopoly of women.

Male nurses are much more likely to rise up the career ladder (Carpenter, 1977, p.180 *passim*). Men's career patterns are not simply or necessarily due to their gender. Men do not take the career breaks which are normal in a woman's working life. Selection criteria are those which favour the continuous male career. In our society, jobs are designed, intentionally and unintentionally, in favour of males. There are insufficient opportunities for part-time working, flexible hours or job sharing. And when men rise to the top in any occupation, the absence of women at the heights demonstrates women's inferior abilities. Thus, in both medicine and nursing, men predominate or are disproportionately represented. As people are prone to appoint others in their own image (Lorber, 1984, p.8), the position of men in both occupations is unlikely to radically change in the foreseeable future.

## The exclusion of women

Why would men want to exclude women? To the extent that their gender contaminates, the presence of women can lower the status of the occupation. Lower status in turn means lower pay. But if gender contaminates, why not appoint women to subordinate positions where they pose no threat to men? Do men prefer the competitive company of other men at work? The evidence from many spheres of activity is that men do prefer to work with other men. Competitiveness and coronaries are to be preferred to the lowering of status which association with women can bring. So it is not surprising to find that women are sidelined and marginalized in so many spheres: in personnel management where women are to be found in the supporting roles (Mackay and Torrington, 1986); in general practice, where women have less chance of finding a partnership (McPherson and Small, 1980); in management, where women – despite being more highly educated than male colleagues – are less likely to be appointed to senior positions in management (Scase and Goffee, 1989); and also in the legal profession, women face an uphill struggle (Dyer, 1991).

In the face of men's antagonism and fear of contamination, women make heroic struggles to establish themselves (Bell, 1953). They make compromises in their career choices and put together 'complicated packages' in order to not to lose touch with medicine (Allen, 1988, p.132; Lester, 1986). Women doctors in particular are dogged in their determination to work and have a higher level of professional activity than other comparable groups such as accountants, architects, or nurses (Doggett, 1988, p.360).

However, the greater willingness of women to accept part-time work means that they are less likely to achieve careers, because questions are then asked about their commitment. If they cannot participate on a full-time basis, workers are extremely unlikely to gain promotion, be offered additional training or enjoy the same financial benefits offered to full-time workers. Women working part-time do so at substantial costs to themselves (Beechey and Perkins, 1987). The contamination which women's gender brings is apparent in the contradictory attitudes to part-time working in medicine. When women work part-time 'it is often seen as failure to utilise fully their state-provided training. For the Consultant, on the other hand, it may be the hallmark of success enabling him (or occasionally her) partially to opt out of the state-funded service' (Elston, 1977a, p.130).

## WOMEN IN MEDICINE

It is no accident that large numbers of women doctors end up in specialties such as psychiatry for which there is relatively little competition for posts. Similarly, areas such as community medicine and radiology attract more than their fair share of women doctors (Allen, 1988, p.246) These are what Stacey (1985, p.284) has called the 'opportunity specialties' where appointments and promotion are easier. These specialties enjoy less prestige, at least in terms of distinction awards (better known as merit awards) which are fewer than in the male-dominated specialties such as surgery (Dowie, 1987); a situation which has not changed much over the years (Leeson and Gray, 1978, p.40). Merit awards mean money, quite a lot of money: anywhere between just under £10 000 to £46 500 each year. It is a privilege worth fighting for. The fight has been relatively successful for male doctors, but women are making some inroads here. Some 20% of female Consultants receive merit awards, compared with 38% of male Consultants (Department of Health, 1992). The specialties in which women are more likely to find senior posts are also likely to offer fewer opportunities for private practice. It is not surprising then that women have been found to do less private work compared with men (Allen, 1988, p.35). Women doctors have been found to be under-represented on all the medical decision- and policy-making bodies (Doggett, 1988, p.337), a situation which perpetuates the disadvantages which women experience.

Women doctors are realistic in choosing the less sought-after specialties. After all, there is no point in choosing a specialty in which you have to fight your way every day of your working life. Women have to fit into the male-dominated occupations where they can (Bradley, 1989, p.70).

Women are marginalized within medicine in other ways. It is women who predominate in the non-career posts within medicine (Doggett, 1988, p.358). Women contaminate an occupation, and reduce that occupation's claims to status. Further contamination takes place through the presence of part-time and casual workers, again reducing an occupation's claim to status. Locum doctors and agency nurses, for example, are viewed less positively in their working practices than their permanent colleagues. From doctors' comments, it is clear they often wish to distance themselves from the activities of their temporary (and often overseas-trained) colleagues.

## MALE–FEMALE RELATIONSHIPS

Most doctors and nurses felt that there was no difference in the relationship between female doctors and nurses compared with male doctors (a similar finding was reported by Heenan, 1991, p.25). Yet quite a few doctors and nurses expressed views about women doctors which reflected some traditional negative stereotypes. Thus women doctors were said to 'get panicky quickly', 'they tend to cry', or 'they can be a bit moody'. (Allen, 1988, p.91, also comments on a similar situation facing female medical students.) The anti-women views among nurses illustrate the status ascribed to medicine and members of the medical profession by nurses.*

For many nurses, doctors are somewhere 'up there'. Doctors are ascribed dominant status and authority because of their association with the magic and special powers of medicine. The dominant-subordinate relationship of doctors and nurses is, in part, tolerated because there is a substantial status-distance between the two. If that status-distance is reduced, say by the presence of women in senior positions, then the status of medicine itself would be questioned. In turn, the subordinate status of nurses would become most uncomfortable. In other words, women doctors disturb the *status quo*. Nurses are noted for their conservatism: they are not world-changers, they are world-menders. They have been reluctant to take up the challenge of feminism. They take pride in their caring and their supportive role. Women who move beyond that role and into the interventionist and decisive role of doctors may be viewed with suspicion.

Women doctors have to tread a fine line between their male colleagues in medicine, and nurses. They must not appear too 'superior' in their relations with nurses, nor must they appear to be over-friendly with nurses to their male colleagues. For women doctors, the contamination of gender can be compounded by the contamination of nurses with lower status. Women doctors must not deny their 'sisterhood' with nurses, but their authority as doctors must not be denied or weakened. They should be able to enjoy 'a good chat', yet not be seen to be merely gossiping. Women doctors occupy an ambiguous position. Among nurses, there was a clear division between those who found women doctors easier to talk to, and those who preferred male doctors because they were uncomfortable receiving directions from women. There was also a division in the ranks of women doctors: over a third of the women doctors interviewed felt they had an easier relationship with nurses, while the rest did not.

* Refer to Ashley (1980).

Among doctors, it always seemed to be someone else who wasn't 'quite sure' about women in medicine. These 'girlies' were sometimes said to become more tearful and emotional. (The words used to refer to women doctors were most revealing; many referring to them as 'girls' or in Scotland, 'girlies'). It is a useful way in which the competence of women can be denied (McAuley, 1987, p.145). The difficulties of combining the roles of doctor and mother, because of the career structures in medicine, were also mentioned.

The implicit and explicit message from some of the nurses' and doctors' comments was that women weren't up to the job: they found it difficult to tolerate the stress, they become more aggressive and bad-tempered. The competition which female doctors posed for nurses to gain the attentions of young male doctors was remarkably salient for some. And the easing of the doctor–nurse relationship which flirty behaviour could bring was notable by its absence.

'I think there's sometimes a little bit of rivalry with women working with women. I prefer working with men. I think that's probably a general reflection. . . . I get on temperamentally better with men than women – I have more men friends than women friends and I sometimes have to work quite hard to get on as well as I do with men.' *Female Consultant*

'A lot of senior doctors still don't regard young women doctors as equals to their male counterparts, but I think that. . . if you were to just look at them across the board, certainly the objective things like exam results and so on, or if they are able to work, if they don't have a family and that they do just as well.' *Senior Registrar*

'You can get a nasty female doctor, worse than the male doctors. . . . Usually they've got real sort of chips on their shoulders in one direction or another.' *Sister*

'I actually prefer working with male doctors than female doctors. . . . I feel more confident with a male doctor than I do with a female doctor. I don't quite know how to explain that, but they often moan a lot more than male doctors, now for whatever reason. Possibly because they have got more to do in their home life, you know, or they are thinking about other things, you know the same way as I would think about what am I going to have for tea tonight or . . . you know I have got things to do. . . . So they tend to, I wouldn't say be lazy, but women doctors I think never are quite as willing to do more than their fair share of work, do you know what I mean?' *Sister*

Female doctors can, however, count on the support from some nurses, and a few women doctors certainly seem to enjoy easier relationships with nurses than their male colleagues. Some 'mothering' of female doctors by female nurses takes place. There is undoubted appreciation among some nurses, particularly the older ones, of the tenacity required from women if they are to succeed in medicine. Alliances are formed between Sisters and women doctors that must act to the disadvantage of male doctors.

It is the attitudes of senior doctors which are likely to be most influential in the careers of women doctors. After all, it is the Consultants who make appointments, who make those off-the-record phone calls, and who act as patrons. It is the all-important informal contacts and the networking from which many women doctors feel they have been excluded (Allen, 1988, pp.165–7). The relative absence of women from senior posts makes the 'networking', which is so useful for medical career advancement, difficult if not impossible. Women's absence from senior positions also means that 'role models' are not available for the young women entering medicine.

## GENDER AND CAREERS

The struggle which women doctors face in establishing a career may be a reflection of a wish to keep women out of the prestigious specialties. If women are kept in the low-status and low-profile specialties, then they can continue to be marginalized within the profession. Medicine can, in this way, continue to be seen as a profession for which men are particularly suited, because it is men who reach the top in the top specialties.

To an extent, the actual gender of female doctors and male nurses is irrelevant. People's gender 'rubs off' on the jobs they do (Cockburn, 1988, p.37). Nursing is a female occupation because women do it. Medicine is a male occupation because men do it. At the same time, because medicine is so heavily involved in science and in being objective and scientific, it is a profession dominated by rationality and suspicious of emotionality. In entering medicine, women must espouse the values of medicine, in turn denying the arguably more female values of emotionality and sensitivity. Women doctors enter a scientific and male world into which they have to adapt. Their femininity is of little assistance in the dominant model of the good clinician. To be good clinicians, women may have to deny their gender and assert the primacy and importance of the dominant (and male) interpretation of medicine.

Women who enter medicine are given 'honorary male' status. To some extent they have to learn to behave like 'one of the boys'. As medical students they may learn to match the beer drinking of their male colleagues; they will be 'buddies' with their colleagues rather than someone to flirt with. They will, as seen in Chapter 3, often look down dismissively on the nurses who seek the attentions of young male doctors.

## Dress and behaviour

As women, doctors have some leeway in the style of dress they adopt. There appears to be little attempt among women doctors to emulate the expensively-cut suit favoured by many male Consultants. With a tendency to eschew high fashion, women doctors also shun trousers. A more casual but distinctive style seems to be most popular, indeed it almost amounts to a uniform. The white blouse, the dark mid-calf length skirt, dark 'flattie' shoes with the white coat on top are favoured by many. There is a need to have some uniformity in dress among members of any occupation. For both male and female it is a means by which a common identity can be established and maintained. It can offer security. The 'uniform' which women doctors wear is not that sported by the thrusting, power-dressing women found in the legal profession, or in the upper realms of business and management. Rather, there is a studied casualness in their dress, reminiscent of that worn by upper-class women when they are doing 'good works'. After all, women doctors are increasingly likely to come from a higher social class than their male colleagues (Allen, 1988, p.54). The woman doctor sporting anything approximating to a working class accent is a very rare bird indeed.

Women doctors are considerably constrained in the behaviour they can adopt. They do not enjoy the same latitude as their male colleagues, women doctors seem to 'get away with' less. As a coping mechanism, flirting is obviously of limited use to them. While they may flirt with male colleagues, some may feel the need to avoid being seen as competition by nurses. At the same time, coquettish behaviour is the behaviour associated with those of subordinate status, not equals (Tellis-Nyak and Tellis-Nyak, 1984, p.1066). The 'giggly' or 'silly' doctor is almost a contradiction in terms, the very antithesis of the serious and professional nature of the job of doctor. Very few women doctors wear make-up, jewellery or high-heeled shoes. They tend not to flaunt their figures, their legs or their looks. Their femininity is not denied, simply not overtly used in a job which is tough and demanding. These women need to be seen as professionals, as competent and certainly not as provoking male comments. Women doctors need also to clearly distance themselves from nurses with their often figure-revealing uniforms.

## The female nurse's uniform

Nurses' uniforms are curious. They actively disable nurses in their work. How can a nurse help lift a patient up the bed in a uniform which 'rides up' when she lifts her arms? Nurses' uniforms make many everyday activities difficult. For Staff Nurses in particular, the uniforms are often thin and reveal what underwear is being worn. Sisters, in their navy blue uniforms, are less transparent. Some nurses obviously enjoy their figure-hugging and short uniforms tailored to show off their physical attributes. Yet for the slightly older nurse the uniform is often unflattering and lacking in style. It is not the sort of thing that would ever be worn off-duty. As well as the colour of the uniform, nurses' belts, badges and hats variously display their status in the nursing hierarchy. The status may not be much apparent to the patients or their visitors, but is carefully noted by colleagues. Hats are a special mark of a nurse's status. By her hat, she can be identified, even in a crowd or from a distance. The hats bear a remarkable similarity, at least at junior nurse level, to those sported by domestic-servants or the waitresses of yesteryear. In some wards and in some hospitals, hats are declining in popularity. Elsewhere a nurse may be dressed 'improperly' without one. Hats are a curious anachronism, to which nurses appear to be attached.

Nurses', or at least female nurses', appearance is very much a gender-defining appearance. Nurses' perceptions of themselves as nurses seem to be closely bound up with their own sense of identity as female. Thus, it would be hard to abandon one without abandoning the other. Nurses' uniforms are obviously part of their occupational identity. It may seem quite reasonable to ask that they wear trousers, like physiotherapists now do, but it could detract from the special connection they make between female and nurse. In picturing nurses wearing trousers rather than dresses, it becomes apparent that nurses would be less identifiably different from others workers. Part of our ideas about nurses in this country is bound up with their uniform, their women's dress. They are not workers like others, but bring a special quality to the work they do, which would be lost if their image were to be redefined.

## The male nurse's uniform

The 'specialness' attached to nurses' uniform is not given to male nurses. In wearing trousers, their male gender is underlined. It would be interesting to know if male nurses are seen as having less of a vocation for nursing by patients, compared with female nurses.

The female doctor can sometimes be mistaken for a nurse, but the male nurse can often be mistaken for a doctor. While the female doctor strives to avoid such a confusion, it seems that male nurses often welcome it. The badge of gender works to produce a lowering of status for the female and an enhancement of status for the male.

'They don't mind going around being called doctor. One man in particular never tells the patient that he's actually the nurse. If the patient says doctor he doesn't say "well actually I'm the nurse". Whereas I would **certainly** contradict them if they . . . frequently say "oh you're the nurse", I'll say "no I'm a doctor".' *Female Senior House Officer*

'I suppose it is a bit sexist but I find, for instance if you go to emergency and there is a male person you assume that they are a doctor, it's easy to distinguish a female doctor from a female nurse, but it's not easy to distinguish a male nurse from a male doctor.' *Senior Registrar*

'But you will find that with male nurses, relatives will talk to them, even male students, they think perhaps he is a doctor or something.' *Registrar*

### Male nurses; career status

Attempts have been made to marginalize male nurses in hospitals: to an extent they have been allotted uncomfortable ground. Just as women doctors are given honorary male status, so male nurses are given 'honorary female' status. The gender of nursing rubs off on the males who do it (Cockburn, 1988). There is a fairly widely-held stereotype of the male nurse being 'gay' or effeminate. The perpetuation of this stereotype acts to marginalize the men who enter nursing. It may also act as a deterrent to men who wish to enter nursing. It is male doctors who were most likely to make connections between homosexuality and male nurses. For some male doctors there was obvious discomfort in having to deal with nurses who were male. This discomfort could come from two sources. Firstly, because of a general fear of homosexuality. And secondly, because it may be more difficult to tell male nurses what to do compared with female nurses. Male nurses, because of their gender, are in a more ambiguous status position than female nurses. The accepted natural dominance of males and subservience of females means that it is easier to control women. If men were to enter nursing in substantial numbers, nursing would offer a greater occupational threat to medicine. It makes sense, in the meantime, for some doctors to counter this threat by attaching the 'gay' label to present and potential male nurses.

A substantial minority of nurses and doctors felt there was no difference in relationships between male and female nurses with doctors (Appendices W and X). Over a quarter of the nurses felt that male nurses had an easier relationship with medical staff. Men are more likely to be listened to, to be assertive, to be treated as 'one of the boys'. Some nurses feel that males are given greater leeway by other nurses: they 'get away with murder', they are 'mothered' and get special treatment from Sisters.

'They [male nurses] seem to be addressed on first name terms from day one, whereas we all get Nurse So-and-so for a while and then the christian name will come in.' *Staff Nurse*

'I think I am even more careful than I am with female nurses not to come across as arrogant, it sounds like a bit chauvinistic thing to say but it is nevertheless the truth.' *Senior House Officer*

'Oh I think there is more of a camaraderie among the male nurses and the doctors, definitely. Oh yes you can see that, even when you go out you know, if you are out for a social evening, and especially if they live in up here, you know they all go to the local, so there is, aye there definitely is.' *Sister*

'I think some doctors are suspicious of male nurses in the same way that nurses are suspicious of female doctors.' *Senior Registrar*

'I find a lot of male nurses . . . the junior ones are more timid than the girls I think, and the senior ones are very aggressive . . . I really do think that male nurses have got an identity crisis when it comes to working with male doctors . . . in terms of power and status.' *Senior House Officer*

Only a small number of doctors actually preferred male nurses (and some of these also preferred male doctors). In nursing, however, there is little doubt that men are more likely to get to the top. Men who have been nurses are particularly well represented in the senior posts within the NHS and even within nursing organizations, such as the Royal College of

Nursing (Owens and Glennerster, 1990, p.39). The dominance of nursing by upper class women is being replaced by a dominance by men (Salvage, 1985, p.9).

Male nurses are more likely to be found in psychiatric nursing, a branch of nursing with a separate history and tradition from general nursing. They tend to be more assertive, partly due, it seems to the nature of the specialty as well as to their gender. For many male nurses, their greater physical size or height may mean that they are not an easy target for ill-humour compared with their female colleagues. In entering nursing, men have made a deliberate career choice which runs counter to those normally considered appropriate for men. Women, on the other hand, who go into nursing are simply choosing a job which is universally seen as appropriate for them. The male nurse may well be more committed that his female colleagues. Male nurses, unlike women doctors, do not appear to find themselves excluded from the prestigious high-tech areas of health care. They do, however, find themselves having a considerable struggle to enter areas which have been completely monopolized by women, such as midwifery.

The camaraderie which exists between some male doctors and male nurses underlines the gender aspect of the traditional nurse-doctor relationship. The male nurses who reach the top in nursing may be more well-disposed to their male Consultants than female nurses. There is evidence from the interviews that a few female senior nurses were less than conciliatory to senior members of the medical profession. (Female doctors were more likely to be given a 'hard time' and have a less easy relationship with nurses in Scotland. Male nurses were more likely to have a less easy relationship with doctors in south-east England.)

> 'Well, one or two have mentioned almost sort of a jealousy among nurses. They're not sure, but they get that feeling there may be some . . . that you know, this fellow female is earning so much more than me, and other things as well.'
> *House Officer*

> 'I think the nurses sometimes, if you are female, they just don't treat you with the same level of respect because they think, because you are a female you are just like them, just the same. I mean that is fair enough but they seem to put

the men up on a higher pedestal.' *Female Senior House Officer*

## GENDER AND STATUS

It seems to be more difficult to deal with discrepancies in status by members of the same gender. Women nurses may find it harder to take orders from women doctors. The similarity in their situations may be more apparent. In other words, differences in status may be more easily accepted in a male-female comparison than in a female-female comparison.

Status discrepancies could be managed by women doctors being friendlier and less 'superior' than male doctors. Thus it seems female doctors are more likely to feel they have an easier relationship with female nurses than their male colleagues. Male nurses, on the other hand, in their relationships with male doctors will handle their status discrepancy either by being more assertive, or by being more friendly. The low-profile is not an obvious choice for the male nurse.

This status discrepancy is of particular interest in considering the strategies of the two occupational groups in relation to one another (see Chapter 11). If alliances are made across occupational lines, then the strength of the dominance exercised by one group is correspondingly weakened. The presence of women in medicine and men in nursing can be interpreted as potentially weakening the disparity in power and status between medicine and nursing. However, if in medicine women are marginalized into the less prestigious roles and specialties then any alteration in the distribution of power will be reduced. In nursing, the 'fast-track' career and the 'honorary female' status of male nurses can also act to minimize any redistribution of power between the two occupations.

If women continue to be numerically superior in the ranks of nurses then there is unlikely to be any substantial change resulting from the presence of male nurses. Any assertiveness or friendliness can be accommodated because it is too infrequent to pose any challenge to the occupational divide. If women doctors continue to be side-lined away from the highly prestigious specialties, then their contribution to policy formation, decision-making and in acting as role models is correspondingly reduced. Any 'softening' of the stance taken towards nursing as an occupation is also likely to be curtailed. In these two spheres, the challenge to the dominance of medicine by nursing can be contained.

# 10

# Graduate nurses

Obtaining academic qualifications is one way in which nurses can challenge doctors on their own territory. Theoretically, it is a way in which the status differences between doctors and nurses can be eroded. If nurses can show that they are academically able, then postures of intellectual superiority can less easily be maintained by members of the medical profession. Only a small number of nurses, however, are graduates with a degree in nursing studies.

## WORKING RELATIONSHIPS

Within nursing, graduate nurses are somehow seen as 'setting themselves above' the traditionally-trained nurses. Just as there is antipathy to women doctors from some women nurses, so there is antipathy towards graduate nurses. Graduate nurses are seen as 'high-fliers', uninterested in ward work, their sights set on advancing up the career ladder (Mackay, 1989). There is, in other words, some feeling among nurses that graduates in some way are a threat to them. Just as women nurses compare themselves unfavourably with women doctors, so they compare themselves with graduate nurses. Again, there is a feeling that these women graduates are challenging the 'natural' male-female relationship and have ideas 'above their station'. At a minimum, graduate nurses often encounter a mixed reception on the wards, and seem to make uncomfortable workmates.

The presence of graduate nurses can be disruptive in that it reminds the non-graduate nurses that they could have followed a different career path. Graduate nurses can also illuminate the lack of confidence and assertiveness in the non-graduate nurses, so assiduously trained out of them. The reception given to graduates within nursing has caused many of them to disguise the fact that they are graduates. The potential challenge to medicine is dissipated by the reception within nursing. One result has been that quite a few doctors and nurses are unaware as to who is, or is not, a graduate. Thus, a potential challenge to doctors from nurses with not dissimilar intellectual qualifications to their own, goes unnoticed.

Graduate nurses also go unnoticed because their numbers are so small. Most nurses and doctors have little or no experience of working with graduate nurses. From the small number of doctors that have had experience of working with graduate nurses, most expressed negative views about them. For these doctors, graduate nurses are believed to lack the practical skills of other nurses. Graduate nurses do have less practical training in that they spend less time on the wards than the non-graduate nurses when training. This of course begs questions about the quality of experience which non-graduate nurses have in their practical training. Counted in on the staffing levels of wards, student nurses are often used simply as another pair of hands, not being trained as such, but merely repeating the same task over and over again (Mackay, 1989).

## Graduate nurses and doctors

A more telling complaint from doctors about graduate nurses is that they are more likely to question doctors' decisions. This was a theme also often mentioned by nurses. This aspect upset some nurses: the accepted roles of doctor and nurse were being challenged. Doctors reported that the graduate nurse was likely to be better informed than her non-graduate colleagues. The repeated emphasis on graduate nurses' poorer practical skills may have been a reminder to graduates not to get too uppity: they were still a long way from being doctors.

Quite a few doctors felt that graduate nurses were to be welcomed and that they had a particular contribution to make to nursing. These doctors may have complained about the lack of initiative among nurses and the refusals to take responsibility. No such comments were made about graduate nurses!

'Well, they seem to be more confident and outgoing and

because they are officially qualified and they've had a spell of experience outside, rather than coming straight into nursing and its closed atmosphere.' *Staff Nurse*

'We're intimidated most definitely, a lot of nurses are. . .' *Staff Nurse*

'They haven't got a very good reputation actually, which is a bit of a shame. The only thing I've ever heard is people sort of scoffing about what they couldn't do on the ward. . . .' *Staff Nurse*

'They have a different relationships with **nurses**. Well, the diploma nurses and degree nurses I worked with – they felt that because they were graduate, I mean diploma or degree, they knew more. But because they hadn't had so much practical work on the wards in actual fact, although they were perhaps third year, a second year normal student knew far more practically and you felt your nose was being put well and truly out of joint. And they'd only perhaps been on the ward once a week and you can't learn. . . . This is a very much practical skill, you can learn all you want in books but in the end of the day it is a very practical skill. . . .' *Staff Nurse*

'They came in and they were getting to do bed pans and they were fed up, they wanted to be able to progress on, and I think most of them could have gone on to be doctors if they'd reorganized their lives properly. And they felt that, and they didn't like it.' *Senior House Officer*

'I think it is good because I think that it gives the nurses more idea that they could be autonomous, and take more responsibility because they are graduates. I found that in the other hospitals we had BA nurses and they were like medical students, they wanted to learn the same things like "will you show me how to do this?" and how to take blood, and "can I watch when you are doing procedures and things?" But the Sisters tended to quite often stamp on them, and go you know "bloody university nurses, they think they know it all", and they were a bit resentful, quite often in fact.' *Senior House Officer*

'Two of the ones that we have had, the medical staff could

not stand, because they felt that the nurses weren't willing to do what they saw as being nursing, and were too willing to interfere with what the medical staff were trying to do, but I agreed with . . . the doctors, because the nurses were trying to interfere in things that they didn't understand themselves, and were too new at the job to understand themselves, and they went about it in rather a tactless way. Having said that, I have had other graduate nurses who have been very good, so maybe it is personalities and who has gone into the graduate course, I don't know.' *Sister*

'I think the main problem that graduate nurses have comes within the nursing ranks, that there seems to me to be reasonably widespread resentment of graduate nurses among non-graduate nurses. I find with the small number of graduate nurses that I have dealt with that some of them are very good indeed, and some of them seem to just have the wrong focus to be a good nurse, what I see as a good nurse. In ICU they are full of information about cardiac physiology and new drugs and things like that, but some of them miss out on the basic nursing stuff.' *Senior Registrar*

'In London, where I did my training, half the people had A levels and the other half had a degree. And one of the doctors said "you've got a degree, what on earth are you doing nursing for?"' *Staff Nurse*

The potential challenge to the medical profession is obvious in comments about graduate nurses really wanting to become doctors and that graduate nurses can be 'a bit superior'. The more negative attitudes towards graduate nurses among doctors may reflect a discomfiture about a potential narrowing of the relative educational distance between nurses and doctors.

## PROJECT 2000

The qualities attributed to graduate nurses, being assertive and challenging doctors' decisions, are those which it is hoped are to be found among the Project 2000 nurses. The United Kingdom Central Council, responsible for setting standards of training for nurses, made recommendations for changes in nurse training which were accepted in 1988. Nurse training is no longer to be undertaken in Schools of Nursing, but in colleges and polytechnics. Student nurses are no longer to be counted in the staffing levels on wards, they are to be 'supernumerary'. Student's 'contribution to service' will also be less than before, with a correspondingly slight decrease in the amount of practical training. (It should be noted that the implementation of the Project 2000 recommendations in Scotland and England has been slightly different.)

Nearly half of the doctors and over a quarter of the nurses felt that the changes in nursing training brought about by Project 2000 were not a good idea (Appendix Y). The effect of Project 2000 on nurse–doctor inter-professional relationships was also investigated (Appendix Y).

Only doctors mentioned that nurses would be unwilling to do 'basic nursing tasks'. Doctors, and to a lesser extent, nurses mentioned the lack of practical experience which these nurses would have. Nurses with their first-hand knowledge of the reality of nurse training on the ward and being used as a 'pair of hands' may be more sceptical about the quality of the practical training that the earlier, non-supernumerary, nurses had received. Yet over a quarter of the nurses asked this question mentioned a reduction in practical skills with the Project 2000 training. Practical skill, after all, is a highly valued component of nursing. Doctors, in also emphasizing the practical skills of nurses, were underlining the value that they place on such skills.

Quite a number of doctors also felt that these new nurses would be more knowledgeable and challenge doctors' decisions – a prospect not always welcomed! Many more negative than positive comments about Project 2000 were made by doctors. Nurses were more enthusiastic about Project 2000, but also guarded in their comments.

There was an undoubted welcoming for the prospect of greater assertiveness and confidence among nurses and for the need to challenge doctors. Nearly a quarter of the nurses felt sure that with the new training, doctors would increasingly come to see nurses as professionals; such a sentiment was rarely mentioned by doctors. The hopes which nurses are pinning of this new training may not be realized, or at least not in the short term, on the wards.

The resentment which the new nurses would encounter was mentioned along with the possibility of having a two-tier structure within nursing. Thus there would be a division between the Project 2000 nurses and nurses who had trained under the previous system.

'Yes I think that in itself – moving them out of schools into colleges and I certainly think the degree nurses are going to earn a lot more respect than . . . because I do think they respect people who do have higher qualifications.' *Staff Nurse*

'They are going to be a lot higher theoretically qualified than we ever were. They will probably be a bit more militant. They will learn a bit more about unionism and what their rights are and I think they will have a bit more confidence to exercise their rights. But they won't be as willing to do the dirty work. They will want to be in on things, which will be resented initially. Because they were just starting this project in Australia when I went there, that's why there was such a shortage of nurses. So I have gone through all they system before. When they first come out to the wards, they are resented like heck. Then everybody starts to realize they are a good thing. They are going to help the image of nursing and they are going to up-lift the opinion of other people outside the whole profession, let alone just doctors, the whole public opinion of nursing. But it just takes a while.' *Staff Nurse*

'Doctors who view nurses with contempt will still do so because they are the kind of people who view anything other than a medical degree with some contempt.' *House Officer*

'I think it's a more gentle introduction to what can be a very harrowing job in some ways, but at the same time I think nursing is a very practical thing, and I think you need to get in early and roll your sleeves up. I think there's a limit to the amount of time you can actually talk about it without actually doing.' *Staff Nurse*

'They will not be as well qualified as doctors, and you would just have to hope that they didn't imagine that they were. It is interesting to see this developing at the time when most of the medical schools are putting more of their medical students back on the wards for their training, it can be very artificial listening to lectures, and reading books without seeing what actually happens at the coal face with the patients. I always feel that learning is best when you have a little hook to hang your knowledge on, the patient with a particular problem that you can read about.' *Consultant*

'Again, I don't really approve of that type of nursing, I am inclined that you know you have to do practical nursing. Again it is the older way of working in the wards, so you actually look after the patients rather than . . .' *Staff Nurse*

'I think that it may well change the way that nurses see themselves, but I don't think that it will change the way that the doctors perceive the role of the nurse. It may make the nurse less willing to occupy the role that the doctor perceives as the nursing role. I think the problem with, if you like, upgrading the sort of perceived educational standard of nurses, I am not talking about their actual education, just what is perceived by both themselves and doctors, that is perhaps more likely to cause confrontation because you start getting the situation where you don't know who is in charge. And I mean there is already enough of a problem with that at the moment.' *Registrar*

'I think nurses won't want to do things like empty bedpans, and they won't feel they should have to care for those sort of needs if they've been to a college.' *Registrar*

The major reservation about the changes in training focused on the reduction in practical skills and experience that newly-qualified nurses would have. Many were also cautious about the emphasis on theoretical knowledge, rather than on the day-to-day work on the wards. But as Delamothe (1988b, p.72) points out: 'What is interesting about the misconceptions of Project 2000 is that they all overestimate its academic standard and scientific content.' This overestimation is apparent from the comments, and may reflect the considerable uncertainty and unease among nurses that they may be downgraded in comparison with the new nurses. The overestimation by doctors may reflect their unease that nurses will increasingly come to challenge their domain, as well as the way in which they work. Knowledge is power and powerful attacks can be made on the medical profession if nurses' knowledge and confidence is increased.

## The impact of Project 2000

The impact of Project 2000 training of nurses had not yet worked its way through the system at the time of the interviews. First-hand experience of the new breed of nurses will undoubtedly affect these opinions. At a minimum, it seems likely that the changes in training will affect the relationship between the two occupations, although this might be a much slower process than anticipated. It will be interesting to monitor what influence the change in nurse training exerts on nurse–doctor relationships.

Another factor which will affect hospitals through the introduction of this new training is the removal of student nurses from inclusion in ward staffing levels. At a time when the population of the UK is ageing and there is a shrinking pool from which to recruit youngsters into nursing, there will be an increased demand for, but a reduced supply of, nurses. The lack of students as 'pairs of hands' on the ward means that more and more work previously done by training and trained nurses will be done by untrained staff. Nurses will increasingly have to spend a greater proportion of their time undertaking technical and skilled work which their unqualified colleagues are not empowered to do. The costs of patient care can thus be reduced. Smaller numbers of qualified, and larger numbers of unqualified nurses, must be the short-term solution to inadequate numbers of nurses on the wards. But short-term solutions could become long-term policy. Nursing will change its shape to become a small, more highly paid elite accompanied by a larger, less well paid rump of unqualified nurses. (A division that is likely to be exacerbated if another recommendation of Project 2000 goes ahead to phase out the auxiliary nurse and replace her by a new category of health care workers who would undergo a brief period of training.) The relationships between nursing and the medical profession will obviously change. Reduced numbers of qualified nurses will mean that nursing may more easily aspire to becoming a profession, and in so doing pose a greater challenge to medicine.

In their relationships with the medical profession, quite a few nurses are of the opinion that everything is fine as it is. They are less happy working with women doctors, with graduate nurses, or with nurses whose training is more distanced from hospitals than their own had been. They accord doctors substantial respect and see no need for change. These are some of the nurses who are not interested in advancing the occupational status of nursing. Their perspective is little different from that of many male doctors. These nurses believe in medicine, in medical science and in the medical model of health care. They believe in it perhaps even more than doctors themselves. They believe in medicine and in hospitals. They believe men should be at the top. They believe that the top people get to the top and the top people are not women. They value men more than women. They will value doctors more than nurses. They will neither appreciate their own nor their nursing colleagues' skills. They will not support their colleagues. They will perpetuate the bitchy atmosphere which is so often found in nursing (Mackay, 1989, Chapter 7). They will value male patients more than female patients (Mackay, 1989, p.146). They even feel that male nurses ought to be at the top. These nurses gain their own sense of value from their association with the dominant group. The dominant group has great value because it is dominant. It is dominant because it is composed primarily of men. That value is reduced when the dominant group is contaminated by women. It is too easy to say that women are their own worst enemies. It might be more correct to say that these nurses are part of the society which accords enormous respect to medicine and medical knowledge. And a society in which the voice of a male carries greater weight and authority than that of women. The awe and deference which the medical profession enjoys is reflected in the everyday experience of these nurses. It would be foolish to expect them to undermine that.

# 11

# A broader look at work and occupations

Many of the complaints of doctors and nurses refer to individual experiences and individual colleagues. Yet at issue is the *relation* of one occupational group to the other. Not surprisingly, each professional group pursues its own interests (Larkin, 1983). The way in which a professional group sees itself and other occupational groups is reflected in the lack of appreciation of the difficulties which members of the other occupation face. It is reflected in views as to how members of the other occupation do behave and ought to behave. These prescriptions and proscriptions are part of a strategy, at times conscious, at times unconscious, to ensure that the interests of one's own occupational grouping are heard and attended to. The dominance of one group involves the derogation of another. It is the way that the occupational pecking-order works. The views of the dominant group will be heard in preference to those of the subordinate group. Greater power, greater pay, greater status will be enjoyed by the dominant group, simply because it is dominant. In many work environments there are dominant and subordinate occupational groups. Whose voice is to be heard, the backroom boys or the front-of-house staff? Whose views are to dominate about the task in hand? What are the factors which play a role in establishing the dominance of one group over another? By looking at the strategies of the two occupational groups concerned with the delivery of health care, many of these factors will be identified.

## MEDICINE AS A PROFESSION

An occupational group can achieve an additional protective status which enhances its potential to dominate other occupational groups, through becoming a profession. For an occupation to establish itself as a profession there are a number of attributes or traits which it is beneficial to possess, such as a body of theoretical knowledge, a 'professional' code of conduct, an emphasis on altruistic service, etc.*

Even though an occupation possesses many of these attributes, it can still fail to establish its claim to be a profession. In part, this failure may be due to the existence, and predominance, of another occupation. Within the organizations concerned with the provision of health care, the medical profession dominates and the nursing 'profession' is dominated. The existence of the medical profession limits the extent to which any claim made by nursing to establish itself as a profession can be successful. Nursing, it seems, must content itself with achieving the status of a 'semi-profession' (Etzioni, 1969).

Medicine, although not one of the original three professions of the army, the church and the law, has become the profession *par excellence*. The ability of medicine to establish, strengthen and maintain its professional position has been an object lesson in strategy, currently under attack. The inability of nursing successfully to establish itself as a profession illustrates many of the constraining factors facing occupational groups seeking to enhance their status.

The label of 'profession' is perhaps the final accolade in the career of an occupation. However, the aspirations of many occupational groups fall far short of professional status. The backroom boys may simply want more recognition of their skills and input, while the front-of-house staff want greater glory and to assert their indispensability. As with many nurses, it is not professional status but respect and appreciation for their skills that is sought. Within nursing, therefore, there is less than wholehearted support for the pursuit of professionalization which senior nurses are pursuing. This division within 'the ranks' of nurses may, arguably, reduce the force of claims for professional status.

---

* An introduction to the issues surrounding professions and professionalization and the arguments surrounding the 'trait' and 'functionalist' approaches is given by Johnson (1972).

## Professions – nursing versus medicine

The history of the two professions is particularly interesting and relevant to the situation today (Abel-Smith, 1960; Bell, 1953; Dingwall *et al.*, 1988; Parry and Parry, 1976). It is a story of move and counter-move by nursing and medicine to establish or maintain their position in the formal system of health care. It is well to remember the inauspicious beginnings as barbers and wet-nurses, when looking at the present-day immaculate occupations of medicine and nursing. The history of both occupations is one of internal divisions and external rivalries.

In the cat-and-mouse game of occupational dominance, the spoils have gone to the medical profession for a number of reasons. There are far more nurses than doctors. It is easier to achieve power and status for small groups than for large groups. Not only is there less possibility of divisions among members but the rewards are also likely to be much greater if entry can be limited. Today, the size of the nursing workforce is well above the critical level that enables governments to relate increases in nurses' pay to increases in income tax. Governments can call forth the dubious shibboleth of 'the national interest' to control nurses' pay. However, the impending shortage of young women from which to recruit nurses also means that the price of nurses may be about to rise (Strong and Robinson, 1988, p.161). The title of 'nurse' is given to unqualified staff such as 'nursing assistant' and 'nursing auxiliary'. The restricted use of the title of doctor, the restricted numbers admitted to medicine and the restricted number of career posts assist doctors' professional status and their dominance.

## Gender and professional status

Gender has been seen as a salient factor in the success of claims to professional status. Nurses have been treated as a disposable workforce within the NHS (Mackay, 1989) and this is related, in part, to their gender. (Within medicine a similar situation is faced by overseas doctors. They too have been seen as a disposable workforce, used to fill posts that home-grown doctors don't want and from which there are limited promotion opportunities. When sufficient numbers of home-grown doctors found posts hard to obtain, language tests were introduced for overseas doctors in order to reduce their numbers (Community Relations Commission, 1976; Smith, 1980). Within medicine, the problems presented by the contaminating gender of women have been managed by encouraging them to enter the less prestigious and less financially rewarding specialties. In this way, the purity of the most prestigious parts of medicine has been maintained by the exclusion of women from senior positions.

The strength of nursing in relation to medicine is not weakened by the presence of men. It does, however, pose a threat to the women within nursing because men rise in nursing, quickly outstripping their female colleagues. The Salmon Report of 1963 in which the benefits of managerialism were extolled, was arguably 'directly favourable to men . . . [and] can be read as an attack upon the effects of female authority' (Carpenter, 1978, p.98). The result has been that men have managed to obtain a disproportionate number of senior positions within nursing (Hardy, 1987). Women nurses' gender is then used against them *within* nursing as well as outside nursing.

In terms of occupational strategy, the predominance of men in the high-status and high-profile specialties of medicine ensures the continuing association between men and success. As long as men can maintain their predominance in the prestigious medical specialties, the gender of nurses can continue to be seen as a negative quality in their struggle for occupational recognition. If, however, women doctors can gain entry in substantial numbers to the prestigious specialties, the gender of nurses may become less important in explanations of occupational subordination. Explanations of dominance may then have to hinge more strongly on class and level of education.

It is interesting to consider whether increased presence of women within the upper reaches of the medical profession will affect the way in which medicine is practised. Some women doctors, such as Young (1981), have suggested that women have distinctive competencies to bring to medicine. To the extent that women doctors can bring a different perspective to bear on medicine, then it may affect the relative positions of nursing and medicine. Whether or not women's distinctive competencies will flower within medicine in the near future is another matter. The strength of the male scientific model of medicine may be just as pervasive as the Nightingale view within nursing.

## LOYALTY

The relative positions of nursing and medicine are controlled by a number of other techniques. For instance, the expectation of 'loyalty' to one's colleagues is one way in which the respective roles of doctor and nurse are reinforced.

'Well my experience has always been that we support each other, even to the extent of covering up.' *Senior Registrar*

'It doesn't matter how bad the doctor is. I know from personal experience that when another ward starts slagging off our team basically, I will jump to their defence.' *Staff Nurse*

Part of the reluctance of nurses to question the decisions of doctors, or indeed to offer their opinions, partly stems from this acceptance of the need for loyalty. It is disloyal to question the doctor. It is not necessary, however, for doctors to publicly demonstrate their faith in the nurses!

As has been seen, quite a number of examples were given where doctors became visibly angry and shouted at nurses in front of patients. It was a cause of considerable embarrassment to nurses if they had been the focus or even a witness to such a public dressing down. The public dressing down, however, can perform a number of different functions. It can act to reinforce the patients' faith in the doctor. It can demonstrate that the doctor wants only the best for his patient and will do anything to ensure that the best is given. It can also demonstrate the power and authority of the medical profession by emphasizing their control over nurses' activities. While nurses may have occasion to tell doctors off, it will not take the form of a public dressing-down.

The public dressing-down can act to underline the ultimate responsibility which members of the medical profession have for their patient. Nurses, trained to be quiescent, will be silent in the face of a public verbal assault. Their subordination to, and domination by, the medical profession will be reaffirmed.

The 'cheeky' nurse who speaks out will incur the wrath of nurses and doctors alike. Nurses will be angry because the patient may come to doubt the efficacy of the treatment being prescribed. Nurses will also be angry because the nurse is speaking 'out of turn'. In the public arena of the ward and the bedside, silence from nurses is golden. The cheeky nurse disturbs the smooth-running and seamless agreement that should be the ward round. The cheeky nurse ensures that the doctor loses face and will have to establish his authority even more forcefully.

## The united front

The need for doctors and nurses to present a united front for the benefit of the patient can, and has been, questioned (Illich, 1977). Perhaps patients should be made aware of the contingent nature of medical knowledge and treatment. Patients' faith in their medical treatment and their subsequent recovery may be affected if the apparent certainty of medical knowledge was questioned. Yet patients cannot make informed decisions if that uncertainty is not revealed. Recovery may be helped if the patient is more committed to the decision taken (Festinger, 1957). The promulgation of loyalty, however, ensures that questioning of medical decisions by nurses and patients is limited. If patients were more sceptical about treatment and outcome, then perhaps patients would seek greater information about, and involvement in, their treatment. Of course, in the process the awe and respect given to medicine and its practitioners would be affected.

Nurses protect 'medicine' and the way it is presented in hospitals from the potentially sceptical eye of the patient. Nurses, despite the assertion of a different view of hospital health care to doctors (see below) have as much invested in the present system as doctors. Less trusting patients are less easy to care for. Instead of being grateful supplicants, the sceptical patient questions and scrutinizes everything. The quiescent patient is a 'good patient', a well-behaved patient for whom it is easy to care. The 'bad patient' is questioning and irreverent of the rules. It is much easier to control the patient who unquestioningly accepts the decisions of doctors and nurses. It is not unreasonable that nurses should do all they can to minimize the possibility that patients will start to question their treatment and care.

The idea of loyalty is deeply embedded in our society. We dislike those who tell tales or who 'grass' on others. We have little sympathy for those who cannot 'hold their tongues'. Yet at issue in every case is some misdemeanour. In every instance, there is likely to be a victim as well as a wrong-doer. Through our notions of loyalty we protect the wrong-doer, not the victim. It is a curious morality. The often-given response of 'it's none of your business' becomes positively immoral when it comes to the care and treatment given to patients. Damage to patients occurs with 'the gradual realisation that 'they' all tell lies and cover up for each other' (Robinson, 1986a, p.35) when there is a complaint. The dominance of the medical profession and the subordination of nursing means that the expectation of loyalty by one from the other will continue.

Loyalty works in the other direction, to a limited extent. Doctors will back nurses if a drug error, as long as it is not too serious, is made. Some mistakes will be overlooked or obscured by doctors in order to protect nurses. These alliances are most likely to take place at junior nurse and doctor level. These are the groups which have to work together on a daily basis and who have to make accommodations to one another. There is less possibility of a stance of self-righteousness being adopted when one is aware that the mistake might just as easily have been one's own. There are the *quid pro quo*s to be honoured, as is the need for the longer-term working relationship to be recognized, plus the need to function collaboratively and cooperatively together in order to provide a reasonable service. It is unrealistic to expect doctors and nurses, especially at a junior level, not to protect one another from blame.

If team-working has not been established, then the possibility exists of each and every mistake becoming common knowledge. It is in these situations that mutual blaming and scapegoating is most likely to take place. Cooperation will be absent. And the question needs to be asked as to whether the absence of loyalty is negative or positive. 'Telling tales' may not mean that the underlying problem is being addressed. It may merely mean that a cover-up takes place further up the hierarchy. Hopes of future cooperation will be reduced and day-to-day relationships become less than easy-going.

Today, a different kind of loyalty is also required of doctors and nurses, that of 'corporate loyalty'. For those who do want to tell tales, who do want to act as whistle-blowers, there is an increasingly hostile reception from the health authority and the hospital. 'Loyalty' is not being asked for, it is being demanded. Jobs will be jeopardized should anyone wish to speak out about standards of care. Talking to the press has become the ultimate crime. Those who finance the NHS, the public, are not to be told when it is failing.

## MISTAKES AND MISDEMEANOURS

There is a difference in the way in which a mistake is dealt with in nursing and in medicine (Strong and Robinson, 1990, p.164). In nursing, the wrongdoer is dealt with through carefully defined procedures. The nurse will be reported to Sister, and then to the Nursing Officer, and if serious enough, to the Director of Nursing. The mistake will be entered in the nurse's personnel record, where it will remain on file for six months, unless it is a mistake for which dismissal is required. Nurses undergo a succession of verbal and written warnings in the event of any mistakes or misdemeanours being made. The primacy of the rules which govern nursing and which so often are the butt of doctors' snide comments are obvious here. The system of control exerted by the nursing hierarchy on nurses working in the clinical area is severe and punitive.

It is a system perfectly designed to foster the covering-up of mistakes. With the prospect of excessive punishment comes the fear of admitting to or reporting the mistakes of others. It is not surprising that in my previous research, some learners mentioned that no one in nursing wanted to hear about bad nursing practices (Mackay, 1989, p.34). There is little doubt that there are bad nursing practices in all specialties. There are good and bad people and good and bad practices in every occupation. In this, nursing, after all, is not so different from other work. Yet there is a failure to confront the lack of support given to nurses reporting mistakes. Within nursing there is a failure to support nurses. Thus nurses exhibit the behaviour of an oppressed group. Conflict within the oppressed takes place because the group is unable to revolt against the oppressor (Roberts, 1983, p.22).

In medicine, the wrongdoer will be subjected to a real 'dressing-down' by his Consultant. Nothing, however, will be written down. The doctor is highly unlikely to be asked to leave. If the mistake is extremely serious then steps may be taken to pursue the matter. Generally, it seems that very few doctors are ever called to account for their actions to the General Medical Council (Robinson, 1986a, p.36). A junior doctor who has made a number of mistakes will find that his reference may be less than glowing. However, that junior will undoubtedly be able to find another post in some particularly downtrodden hospital in an area which normally has difficulty attracting any junior doctors. The unrecorded misdemeanours will not follow the doctor throughout his career. Once made and remonstrated over, the mistakes can be more or less forgotten, unless of course, the patient sues or a complaint is accepted by the General Medical Council.

Throughout medical training there is a golden rule imprinted on the minds of all prospective doctors: **You Must Not Criticize a Medical Colleague**. Doctors' individual practices are very seldom commented on by other doctors (at least to those outside the profession). Doctors also may be circumspect in what they say to colleagues (Young, 1981, p.150). Members of the medical profession can count on the silence of their colleagues. They will not be judged and they will not be censured unless there is evidence of grave misconduct. Grave misconduct will encompass criminal activity, excessive drug and alcohol misuse as well as ethical issues such as euthanasia. Very, very few doctors are struck off the register of the General Medical Council each year. Doctors look after their own, unlike nurses.

## Keeping silent

The silence of the medical profession has been a source of its strength. There are good reasons for protecting individual doctors from the whimsical complaints of patients and for uninformed comments from colleagues in other specialties. Yet within a hospital and within a specialty, doctors will be aware of the disparity in the performance of say, two surgeons. One surgeon's operations may have a much higher success rate than the other's. There may be a number of reasons for the difference in performance: the type of patients, catchment area, differing prognoses, etc. Yet poor practices will not be commented on* and the unsuspecting patient will be unable to avoid being operated on by the inferior surgeon.†

Doctors may name 'the best man in the field' to friends, but a variation in competence at an everyday level will not be admitted. Some measure of protection may be afforded by general practitioners in their referrals to particular hospitals or Consultants. The recent introduction of medical audit will mean that the medical profession will be subjected to a degree of scrutiny by their peers. Although the findings of any audit will not be made public, the wall of silence and secrecy has at least been breached.

In nursing, the incompetence of nurses will only too readily be admitted. Their public punishment by senior nurses and the marking of their records makes it clear that misdemeanours will not be tolerated. Nursing polices its own members in order that no one else will feel the need to do so. Coser (1972, pp.183–4) points out that, 'Nurses are often in a position in which the insistence on rules serves as a means to assert themselves and to display some degree of power.' Nursing, in disciplining its own members, can quickly stifle any attempts by members of the medical profession to criticize nursing practice. Nursing's toughness in dealing with wrong-doers reflects its position of relative weakness in comparison with medicine.

The pursuit of wrongdoers within nursing has meant, as already mentioned, that nurses incline to silence rather than speak out about bad nursing practices. (The reception given to 'whistle-blowers' within the NHS is not a warm one. The Graham Pink affair is the most recent example of a nurse being blamed for the quality of care being tolerated within some parts of the NHS, in his case the care of the elderly). The career victimization which takes places acts very efficiently to intimidate others who might consider speaking out. It is the

---

*    Millman (1976, p.10) discusses this with regard to the USA.
†    Reeve (1980, p.567) reports that according to his stability index of behaviour, 20% of Consultants he studied may represent a risk.

message rather than the messenger which ought to receive attention (Robinson, 1986a, p.36). Whistle-blowers within the medical profession are also dealt with harshly, as in the case of Helen Zeitlin, the haematologist who spoke out about her hospital becoming a trust (Phillips, 1991). The fact that Pink was a male nurse and Zeitlin a female doctor may be incidental, but it is worth noting. Martin (1984, p.246) points out that it is the marginal people in organizations who are most likely to speak out. It seems that nurses also frequently fail to speak out about what they perceive to bad medical practices, particularly in the case of the terminally ill patient. Perhaps these two areas of silence are linked. It must be easy once one has learned to hold one's tongue about bad nursing to do the same for bad medicine.

The strategy to protect the occupation of nursing from outside censure also acts to weaken its claims to a professional and independent practitioner role within the provision of health care. The patient is left without a defender because the occupation is defending itself.

## DIVISIONS WITHIN OCCUPATIONS

Occupational defence at the expense of the patient is also encountered when there is conflict between doctors. It is a mark of the strength of the medical profession that the public expressions of diverging views can, for the most part, be contained (although the recent divisions within medicine about junior doctors' hours demonstrated that the medical profession does not always publicly present a united front). The failure of nursing to establish such a common front is one of its occupational weaknesses. Not only are there divisions caused by the lack of support given to one nurse by another, but there are also divisions due to occupational ideology. Some of the reasons for this have been given above. The rule-dominated behaviour and the emphasis on discipline has acted to divide, rather than unite, nurses. (For a discussion of the effects of this on nurses, see Mackay, 1989, Chapter 7).

Despite the publicly presented front of the medical profession, there are divisions within the ranks of doctors in their day-to-day working. The presence of these divisions is not mentioned without prompting. Conflicts and difficulties between medical colleagues are a predictable and natural part of hospital life. These conflicts can affect inter-professional relations. Nurses are often dragged into squabbles between doctors and they have to be very careful not to align themselves with one or the other too clearly.

## Autonomy and independence

Doctors are trained to work on their own. They are trained to rely on their own, independent judgement. They need and enjoy autonomy in their clinical decision-making. The issue of clinical autonomy is fundamental to the position of dominance of the medical profession (Elston, 1977b, p. 27) and why the introduction of medical audit is so significant. Doctors, so it is argued, must be free from any constraint in deciding what treatment is appropriate for their patient. This means that the individual rights of each doctor are supported, no matter what (Strong and Robinson, 1990, p.35). The notion of clinical autonomy is also used to explain why misdemeanours may not be pursued. As Smith (1987b, p.1583) points out, it can be used as a 'glib excuse occasionally put forward to explain why the profession does nothing about behaviour that is, in reality, inexcusable.' This autonomy and independence within the ranks of medical practitioners means that a great deal of idiosyncratic behaviour is tolerated and expressions of individuality are both expected and appreciated. For a substantial part of the time, doctors work in relative isolation from their colleagues (Green, 1974, p.67) and the opportunity for any conflict is correspondingly diminished. To the extent that senior doctors work in a team, they tend to see themselves as heading that team. It is not as collaborators but as leaders that doctors identify themselves. This in turn casts doubt on the ability of doctors to operate on a group basis (Green, 1974, p.105). However, at the more junior levels such independence is not possible; junior doctors work as members of a medical 'team' in which they enjoy little autonomy. Because of this, there are likely to be conflicts with colleagues on a regular basis. For the junior doctor, working with other House Officers there are all the usual working problems of personality conflicts, individual competitiveness as well as differences of personal style and behaviour, bickerings over rotas, complaints of tasks left undone for others to do and complaints about sloppy practices. Further up the ladder, competition becomes much more cut-throat. According to many doctors, a doctor has to be tough to survive in hospital medicine. As a Registrar, despite the years of experience one is constrained by the practices of one's seniors. One has to 'look good' for that valued Senior Registrar's post and it is not advisable to cross the path of your Consultant. The constraints of the system of hospital medical careers ensures that it is only at Consultant level that the valued independence and autonomy can fully be enjoyed. (That autonomy is being challenged today by the ever-present constraints of budgetary control.) Even at Cor ,ultant level, there can be feuds between mismatched colleagues who may refuse to speak to one another for years. Personal animosities may mean that one Consultant refuses to refer any of his patients to a disliked colleague. One Consultant may take every possible opportunity to irritate the other, or to score points off him. Another particularly ambitious Consultant may ensure the ascendancy of his specialty at the expense of colleagues in other specialties. (There are, of course, also status differences within medicine: the status of the hospital, level of research activity, amount of private practice among others, will reflect status differences (Green, 1974, p.66). Such difficulties are to be found in every hospital. Bound by professional standards of behaviour the frustrations of working with intolerant and intolerable colleagues can obviously be substantial yet remain unvoiced.

### Disputes

At a clinical level there can also be disputes between doctors. For example, anaesthetists with a thorough understanding of intensive care may disagree about the treatment suggested by the surgeon whose only wish is to save the patient and who refuses to give up on the patient. Occasionally, patients can be under the joint care of two Consultants which can obviously result in differences of opinion. And although the admitting doctor has ultimate responsibility for the treatment of the patient, this does not dispose of the problem of disagreements about treatment.

There is reluctance to discuss the presence of conflict between doctors but when asked, many respondents did comment on its presence. It is obvious that such conflict can, like any other occupational conflict in health care, affect the patient. Tensions between doctors may mean that there is delay in reaching decisions. Personal squabbles may mean the best opinion is not sought, or that one course of action is pursued because of pigheadedness rather than careful deliberation. None of these situations is surprising. Indeed, it would be more surprising if there were **not** such conflicts. Yet the role of nurses in this intra-professional conflict is revealing.

## The role of nurses in doctor disputes

Nurses are much involved in doctor–doctor conflict. Indeed, they often have to manage that conflict in order to obtain a clear decision about patient management. Nurses may be particularly supportive of one doctor who is being given a hard time by another. Nurses disguise the presence of conflict between doctors, just as they disguise the presence of conflict between nurse and doctor. The 'not-in-front-of-the-patient' rule is brought into play. The patient is 'protected' from the knowledge that there is disagreement between doctors, just as the patient is protected from awareness of disagreement between nurse and doctor. The united front which the medical profession wishes to purvey is not likely to be dented by nurses.

Being privy to the secrets of doctors places nurses in a potentially powerful, yet also invidious, position. Occupying a place in the middle of a conflict between two doctors is difficult when those doctors have substantially more power than the nurse. Diplomacy is the order of the day. If nurses do not manage their role in the middle they can end up being blamed for the actions of the other. Nurses' relative lack of power means that they have to protect the interests of the more powerful medical profession in order to maintain the image of a united front.

In both medicine and nursing, the occupations appear to look after their own interests, even though these may be at the expense of the patient. It is not surprising to find such strategies within an occupation. We don't realistically expect the car mechanic to admit he made a mistake in the wiring which later caused the engine to go on fire. We don't realistically expect a social worker to admit his failure to recognize the signs of violence in a family. We don't expect the water authority to admit it is responsible for a major polluting incident. We expect them to be economical with the truth. And we expect occupations will have developed strategies to protect themselves. Those strategies will include the development of protective services from trade associations, trade unions, professional bodies, etc. Doctors have been described as having one of the best trade unions in the world (Strong and Robinson, 1990, p.39) against which the RCN contrasts vividly.*

Uncertain in its role, with huge numbers of members and affiliated members, it lacks the clout, influence or power of the BMA. All the weaknesses of nursing, in contrast to medicine, are reflected in the muscle of the professional bodies.†

(It is interesting to consider the change in the fortunes of the RCN which might accompany the Project 2000; changes to the extent that an elite and a rump of nurses are formed. It could mean that the membership of the RCN sharply declines while that of the trade unions correspondingly increases. In turn, the willingness of the new 'helpers' in health care to take industrial action may be greater than that of nurses.)

### Protective strategies

The extent to which an occupation has developed protective strategies is likely to reflect its position in the occupational pecking order. Whether an occupation is a fully-fledged profession, as in the case of medicine, or a semi-profession, as in the case of nursing, reflects its ability to look after its members' interests, and not those to whom their services are rendered. Although associations have been formed to protect the interests of clients, consumers and patients, these associa-

---

* Berlant (1975) also discusses professional bodies in medicine.
† It is worth noting that both the General Nursing Council and the General Medical Council have representatives from the other occupation on their Council, appointed as lay members, rather than as members of nursing or the medical profession, by the Secretary of State.

tions are always less strong than the occupational bodies. Occupations tend to look after themselves: their jobs and their interests always come before those of their clients. Occupations set up structure through which they look after themselves, while the client is accorded a lower priority than their members' interests.

## THE CONFIDENCE GAME

Nurses do not give themselves sufficient respect. This is a recurring theme. The nurse puts the doctor on a pedestal and implicitly places herself at some lower level. The acceptance of that difference in level, prevents an equal exchange of information. Communication too easily becomes one-way. Silence and acquiescence becomes the accepted stance for nurses to adopt. There are some doctors who quite clearly like it that way. Their decisions are not questioned and perhaps the need to reflect on or question their own practice is avoided. It is a way in which self-doubt can be ignored and confidence retained. Nurses' silence is of use to doctors.

### Confidence levels

It is curious that there is so much complaint from nurses about the 'confidence game' played by doctors when their own behaviour exacerbates it. The confidence game relates to behaviour by doctors known as the 'Great-I-Am'. It is an affliction most noticed among junior doctors. Newly propelled into hospital practice from medical school, House Officers are keenly aware of their lack of experience. These pre-registration House Officers having ostensibly 'completed' their training, can be chastened by the extent of their ignorance when they arrive on the wards. The response of some is not to admit to that ignorance. In pretending to have confidence, the young House Officer hopes to pass muster, to be seen to know what he is doing. As a medical student, he will have closely monitored the behaviour of qualified doctors; he will have perhaps modelled himself on one such doctor. He has learned to behave in a way that seems appropriate as a member of the medical profession. It is only to be expected that some doctors get it wrong and overdo the expression of confidence. For other doctors, the assumption of clinical responsibilities is accompanied by *arrogance*. It is an unattractive quality to encounter in anyone and it is not surprising that nurses take particular issue with it.

However, the arrogant doctor is often a doctor lacking in confidence. Yet the doctor must feign a confidence he does not feel. Nurses expect doctors to take decisions. Nurses, especially the more junior and less experienced, expect speed and confidence from junior doctors in their decision-making. The doctor's behaviour is being affected and moulded by the nurses' expectations. Just as in the 'doctor-nurse game', where nurses disguise their greater knowledge in helping doctors to look good in front of patients, so there is a counter-game being played.

This behaviour is intriguing in that it is so often tied up with negative perceptions of nurses. Thus it appears that doctors who need to assert their dominant position, simultaneously feel the need to be disdainful towards nurses. It is a way in which one occupational group can distance itself from another and at the same time, denigrate any attempts to make the relationship more equal. The 'Great-I-Am' behaviour serves a useful purpose. Any attempts by nurses to establish their own distinctive areas of competence or view of health care will more easily be rubbished by doctors if they are able to feel they are greatly superior to nurses.

The 'everyday-ness' of the tasks that nurses do has ensured that their work is seen as neither distinctive nor skilful. At times there has been little to distinguish nurses' activities from those of domestics or nursing auxiliaries. If nursing is to establish itself as worthy of professional status, it needs to define its own specific and identifiable role. Indeed, if it does not, others will do so for it (Mills, 1983, p.5). Within nursing, a number of strategies have been used in an attempt to define that special role.

## THE PATIENT'S ADVOCATE

Patients find it hard to say what they feel to doctors; they may not know their rights and it may be difficult to make decisions. As the patient's advocate the nurse will ensure that the patient can make an informed decision. They will act as a 'go-between', communicating the wishes of the patient to the doctor and ensuring that the patient's interests are safe-guarded (Castledine, 1981, p.40). Nurses will act as inter-mediaries between the doctor and the patient, interpreting and conveying information. This potentially establishes nurses as a critical lynch-pin in the health care team. It is not clear that the patient's advocate role is realizable or that nurses have been suitably trained to adopt such a role (Castledine, 1981, p.40). In the care of the terminally ill, nurses' reticence in speaking out on behalf of the patient, points to the difficulties in becoming the patient's advocate. There is a danger, also, that nurses come to adopt a position on the moral high-ground. In other words, that nurses *know* what patients want, whereas doctors do not and cannot know. The implicit attempt to exclude or squeeze out doctors from an intimate com-munication with patients is suspect. While it cannot be doubted that the patients' wishes and views must be taken into account, to limit the expression of those views to one channel is dangerous. The patient should be of central concern to all those involved in health care. The attempt should be made to ensure that maximum possible communication with the patient takes place, and not simply a restricted dialogue.

### Patient contact

Seldom mentioned in relation to the patient's advocate role of the nurse is the lack of contact that qualified nurses have with patients. (The amount of patient contact which nurses have will, of course, vary from specialty to specialty. Qualified nurses in ITU for example will have a great deal of patient contact, while their colleagues in general surgical wards will have much less.) Patients have their everyday needs attended to by untrained and unqualified nurses. It is the domestics or the nursing auxiliaries who run little errands which make life tolerable on the ward. It is not the Staff Nurse who helps you wash yourself. You seldom have a chat with Sister: Sister comes and looks at all the patients, reads your notes, nods and walks on just like the Consultant. Staffing levels on wards don't allow the trained nurses to spend their time in such a frivolous activity as talking to patients. They are too expensive. They have much to organize and to arrange; great piles of paperwork to plod through and people to manage. The hands-on part of nursing soon recedes into memory for the nurse who has been qualified for a couple of years. The medical profession wants nurses' knowledge of the patient, yet that knowledge is often little more than that acquired through the patient's notes. That is the knowledge that doctors want and value, therefore that is what nurses pretend to give. Just as with the care of the dying, the medical profession sets the agenda. Nurses are losing touch with the patients. Maybe some want to, others certainly do not. Yet there is a pretence that nurses spend their time with patients: they simply haven't time to do that any more.

The abdication of the medical profession from patient 'care' has meant that they do not listen to their patients, or rather they do not listen to what is **not** said by their patients. In delegating this role to nursing staff, the assumption has been made that nurses have the time to perform this function. Reductions in nurse staffing levels have proceeded apace over the years. Occasionally, stout defences on behalf of staffing levels are made by senior doctors, though too often those defences are simply made with a view to maintaining patient throughput. The quality of patient care given by nurses has not been evaluated. Re-admission rates do not tell you how well a patient was treated; how considerately or how patiently they were dealt with. What is happening to patient care? Would you want to be a patient today?

Many of these occupational strategies have been undertaken at the expense of patients. Doctors and nurses have been fighting for territory. There is little doubt that there are grave disparities in the amount of territory enjoyed by nurses and doctors. Yet at the same time, this fighting has not been in the patient's interest. Doctors and nurses often seem to see their own jobs first and the service they provide for patients, second. Professions become an end in themselves. Is that what nursing wants to become?

The patient certainly seems to be in need of an advocate. It is not clear that nurses are in a position to provide that role. And it is not clear that doctors would have any interest in that role being provided.

## Graduate nurses

The introduction of graduates into hospital nursing can be seen as another occupational strategy to increase the respect given to nurses by the medical profession. As has been seen, it has met with only limited success and there is some antagonism towards graduate nurses from within the ranks of nursing. At the same time, some doctors are less than enthusiastic about graduate nurses. Doctors' comments that such nurses really wanted to become doctors perhaps illustrate the threat which graduate nurses might pose.

## THE SPECIALIST PRACTITIONER

Another attempt to counter the unequal relationship has been that associated with the idea of the nurse as an 'independent' or 'specialist practitioner'. This idea was seldom mentioned in the course of the interviews without prompting. The nurse practitioner would be highly trained in her own specialty and able to offer advice to less-trained colleagues. She will practise with skill and judgement, and be responsible for her own actions. She will develop the role of acting as consultant to other nurses as do, for example, stoma care nurses and diabetic nurses. The presence of such nurses has, by and large, been accepted by the medical profession. It is useful, for instance, if a diabetic nurse can be brought in to advise a patient on diet and injecting themselves. The doctor is relieved of a time-consuming activity and one which does not enjoy great kudos among hospital doctors. The idea of the specialist practitioner accompanied the recommendations of Project 2000, the UKCC's proposals for the development of nursing into the 21st century. The idea has enjoyed particular favour with the group within nursing which wishes to pursue the path of professionalization.

## NURSE TRAINING

Those who wish nursing to become a profession achieved a notable success when the recommendations of Project 2000 were implemented (Chapter 9). Some of the impetus to altering nurse training undoubtedly was a response to the jibes of members of the medical profession (Clark, 1984, p.49). With nurse training more firmly situated in the realms of higher education, it is hoped that nursing will enjoy greater status and be accorded greater respect – especially by the medical profession.

The general response to the changes brought about through Project 2000 is somewhat mixed. It was primarily nurses and only a tiny proportion of doctors who felt that Project 2000 training of nurses would foster doctors' awareness of nurses as professionals. It seems, at this stage anyway, that this nursing strategy to overcome the inequality in the doctor-nurse occupational relationship is not going to meet with un-qualified or immediate success.

### THE EXTENDED ROLE

Another strategy which the nursing profession has used to overcome the imbalances in the doctor-nurse relationship has been to more clearly define the division of labour between nurses and doctors. This has been achieved through the introduction of a rule that nurses need to possess an extended role certificate in order to perform certain tasks. The tasks are those which are associated more with the duties of the medical profession than with nursing, such as the administration of intravenous drugs, taking blood samples, doing ECGs (electro-cardiograms).

Most of the tasks covered by the extended role certificate are those which many members of the medical profession feel that nurses should perform. Doctors as an occupational group are keen to divest themselves of tasks which they now feel to be onerous. (And if doctors can delegate their routine tasks to nurses they can keep the numbers of recruits to medicine low, their earnings high and increase their professional domain, according to Gardner and McCoppin, 1986, p.26). Nurses as an occupational group have responded, until recently, by restrict-ing the ease with which such tasks can be re-allocated to nurses. The seriousness of the tasks which doctors are seeking to hand over to nurses is being emphasized by the need to take the extended role certificate. The stance taken by senior nurses has been double-edged in its effects. Nurses must receive training in order to carry out these tasks, while doctors needed no such training or certification. The impetus to the introduction of the extended role certificate may have been to assert the ability of nursing to establish and maintain a high level of safe practice among its members. At the same time, nursing may also have underlined the difference in ability between doctors and nurses. There is one rule for doctors and another for nurses. The presence of yet another set of rules within nursing has been greeted by some doctors with ridicule. After all, many nurses were previously administering IVs and taking blood samples without the need for a certificate. These same nurses now have to take that certificate before they can perform tasks which they may have done for years.

The tasks covered by the extended role certificate cause particular frustrations to members of the medical profession. It is no accident that nursing has responded in such a way. The division between the occupational groups has been defined and clarified. The need for the certificate means that doctors cannot just dump unwanted tasks onto nurses. The division of labour between the two occupations has always been in a state of flux. It is not so long ago that nurses were not allowed (by the medical profession) to take blood pressures. That task now is an accepted part of nursing activity. Because nursing is aspiring to achieve some equivalence with the medical profession it must increasingly be in control of determining the nature of nursing work. If such determination is left to another occupational group, then professional status will never be achieved. The refusal to allow doctors to pass on unwanted tasks to nurses has also meant that nursing has an increasing role in deciding which tasks doctors should perform. The BMA (1981, p.42) makes its own position clear: it wants to continue to be able to delegate tasks: 'it has no desire either to restrain the delegation to such persons of treatment or procedures falling within the proper scope of their skills. . . .'

This occupational strategy within nursing has, to some extent, worked. There is an acceptance of the division of labour by the medical profession and the ability of nursing to determine its own role has been established. The success of this strategy is not liked by many within medicine. In the interviews with doctors, the 'nursing hierarchy' was repeatedly blamed for restricting the tasks that nurses can do. Some nurses were seen, by doctors, as wanting to do more (Appendix Z).

This was corroborated by over 60% of (the admittedly limited number of) nurses who were asked about the nurses' role. The wish of nurses to increase their role is only temporarily impeded by the need to have an extended role certificate. The underlying success is that any change in nurses' roles will be at the discretion of those in charge of nursing, and not those in charge of medicine, although this situation is now in the process of changing. The introduction of clinical directorates, the increasing emphasis on budgets and medical audit will all affect what tasks nurses are to do and decisions will not necessarily be made by nurses.

The recent agreements to reduce junior doctors' hours will provide an excellent opportunity for the medical profession to pursue its own occupational strategies. Because of the reduction in junior doctors' hours and, by extension, of the amount of work they can do, additional pressure will be exerted on nurses to undertake some of the tasks currently undertaken by junior doctors. At the moment there appears to be considerable sympathy among nurses for the pressures under which junior doctors work. However, the reduction in their hours, no matter how small, is likely to reduce nurses' sympathy if nurses are being pressured to do additional tasks. The long-standing debates surrounding the division of labour between doctors and nurses are set to continue.

It is important to note that there are local differences in the stance taken by senior nurses in different locations regarding the extended role. In some hospitals, the extended role of the nurse seems to be accepted practice. In other hospitals, it appears that there is a reluctance to release nurses in order to let them attend the accreditation course. Pressures on nurse staffing levels were one of the reasons given for limiting the numbers taking the extended role certificate. In some areas, it seemed that the nursing hierarchy was not only unenthusiastic about nurses taking the certificate, but there was also a reluctance to let nurses perform those tasks even when they had obtained their certificate. A small minority of nurses expressed frustration at being denied a greater role. The presence of this group, however, points to a division within nursing as to the direction in which nursing as an occupational group should be progressing. The occupational strategies adopted within nursing do not enjoy universal support. Similarly, ideas regarding the appropriate direction for nursing to proceed, change. It now appears that support for the idea of the extended role is weakening within the UKCC (1991, p.7) because the boundary practice implied in the extended role 'may unduly limit practice to the disadvantage of patients and clients and prevent practitioners from fulfilling their potential.'

## THE PROFESSIONAL AGENDA

The group of nurses seeking to establish nursing as a profession is to be found primarily in the field of nurse education (Melia, 1984, 1987). This 'professionalizing' group of nurses is currently in the ascendancy within the occupation (Robinson, 1986b). Nevertheless, there is an influential and vocal group of nurses which is concerned that qualified nurses should not distance themselves too greatly from their unqualified colleagues. Many commentators have voiced concerns about the dangers of professionalizing and creating two tiers within nursing (Ehrenreich and English, 1973; Leeson and Gray, 1973; Mackay, 1989; Melia, 1987; Salvage, 1985). Nurses in this group would wish to emphasize the common concern of nursing auxiliaries and qualified nurses: that of caring for patients through the range of duties from giving out bedpans to planning pain control. The 'dirty work' is an important part of nursing and in trying to pass this on to unqualified and untrained staff, the nurse will be creating a distance between her and the patient (Johnson, 1978, pp.112-3). The professionalizing group within nursing would seek to more closely establish its links with the medical profession by losing the 'dirty' work. Hanging onto the coat-tails of medicine, nursing could become a highly skilled and specialist occupation, technically competent, although limited in numbers. If the numbers of nurses can be reduced, then nursing can become and be seen as a scarce, and therefore more valued, occupational group. The creation of a profession means an elite and a rump. The 'rump' would comprise all those involved in the provision of health care who are unqualified and untrained. The elite would perform a role more akin to that of an assistant doctor than that of a nurse. The elevation of a few would be achieved at the expense of the majority of nurses, consigned to low-status and low-paid work. As Dingwall (1988, p.227) notes, 'Throughout the occupation's history a professional segment has sought to squeeze out the handywoman class from the care of the sick. . . . .they have sought to gentrify the plot of work owned by the occupation.'

Differing opinions as to the 'proper' role of the nurse provide an additional division within nursing. In the view of the professionalizer, nursing can and should take on highly technical tasks and act as a specialist practitioner (hence the argument that the professionalizers have 'won the day' in the acceptance of the recommendations of Project 2000 regarding the specialist practitioner; Robinson, 1986b). This nurse will take on tasks previously performed by doctors and also undertake tasks similar to those currently being performed by doctors. For example, the 'professional' nurse could strip veins in preparation for the performance of heart by-pass surgery (Illman, 1989). The anti-professionalizing group within nursing identifies separate roles for nurses and doctors. (This is not to deny that the two occupations could collaborate or work in harmony.) This group of nurses is concerned with the provision of 'nursing care' and feel nurses have a sufficiently wide role not to need the addition of any cast-off medical tasks. In this view, helping someone go to the toilet is just as important as doing an ECG. These nurses see the need for nursing to have as its goal a more professional approach, but not with all the trappings of 'a profession', which would seek to exclude un-qualified nursing colleagues. These nurses, and they were often some of the most committed, did not want to take on extended role duties or to increase the amount of 'technical' nursing.

The occupational strategies within nursing will be weak-ened by the presence of diverging views. There are nurses, particularly in specialties such as intensive care, who are keen to expand their knowledge and skills in technical and medical areas. These are the nurses who can be seen as aspiring to become 'assistant doctors', although they may not necessarily wish to abandon their caring role. There are other nurses who are keen to develop the caring skills of nurses and to act as a counter to the perspective of the medical profession. This division is, of course, a simplification. The divisions are not as clear-cut or as straightforward. Nevertheless, the tensions within nursing means that advances towards professionalization are being resisted.

## DIFFERING 'WORLDVIEWS'

The assertions made by nurses that they have a different 'worldview' from their medical colleagues is another occupational strategy used to distance nursing from medicine. Nurses, so they argue, take an holistic view of the patient while doctors adopt a curative- and disease-oriented perspective of the patient. Thus while doctors focus on the disease, nurses focus on the illness (Campbell-Heider and Pollock, 1987, p.422). Undoubtedly there is strength in nurses' claims that they do try to take a different view of the patient. After all, nurses are ward-based and have the opportunity for greater personal interaction with patients than do their medical counterparts. There is also little doubt that nurses in general have more highly tuned inter-personal skills than doctors. The claims regarding the differing worldviews, however, are easily translated into 'better' and 'worse' views of the patient. It simply depends on where you stand. If you are a patient with peritonitis you're not terribly concerned with the social skills of your doctor, but you are concerned about the correct diagnosis being made and effective treatment of your condition. A mastectomy patient learning to adjust to the loss of her breast will be more concerned with the support and sensitivity of the nurses. Different patients make different demands on the various members of the health care team. One worldview is not superior to another, merely different.

It is only relatively recently that nurses have sought to establish a discrete worldview regarding health care. Not so long ago, nurses were reprimanded if they were seen to be chattering to the patients and being too familiar. Such a view has long roots within nursing (Carpenter, 1977, p.166). Johnson (1978, p.122) has commented that, '. . .cleaning out the sluice room was in times past a common punishment for juniors who were caught in the worthless act of talking to patients.' The present emphasis is on the need for interpersonal and social skills in dealing with patients. This worldview has been successfully adopted within nursing. Today the nurse is taught to be concerned with the emotional and social, as well as the physical needs of patients. The majority of nurses will be appreciative and supportive of the need to offer such support to patients. Nursing is building its own ideology on which to more firmly base its claims to professional status. The need now is for nurses to demonstrate that the existence of a different view of health care can positively affect patient care and recovery. To the extent that this goal can be realized, then the specific contribution which nurses have to make can be more clearly recognised.

## THE NURSING PROCESS

Part of the changing view of nursing is encapsulated in the introduction of a new way of nursing: the nursing process. Introduced in response to the demands of nurses rather than with addressing patients' needs (Dingwall *et al.*, 1988, p.214), the nursing process has enjoyed considerable success in the UK. Instead of a nurse performing a specific task for all patients in the ward, under the nursing process the nurse is allocated to only a few patients. The patient is to be treated as a whole person rather than simply an object which requires that certain tasks be performed for it. The nurse is to make her own 'care plans' for each patient, detailing the care that the patient had received, and was to receive. The fragmentation of the task-centred approach was replaced by a concern for the well-being of individual patients to whom the nurse was assigned.

The nursing process has come in for substantial criticism. The nurse's care plans over-emphasize medical tasks and physical care and the need for documentation can result in an intrusive interest regarding patients' personal lives (Armstrong, 1983, p.458; Lawler, 1991, p.216). When staff are short in number, a priority was shown for physical care and still 'talking is not regarded, either by the nurse or by her superiors and peers, as doing something useful for the patient' (De la Cuesta, 1983, p.369). According to Lawler (1991, p.36), this was part of an attempt to 'scientise' nursing.

Nursing can be seen to have been successful in challenging

the medical profession through the introduction of the nursing process. The medical profession did not like it and it was seen as part of 'the progressive exclusion of doctors from nursing affairs' (Mitchell, 1984, p.29). The nursing process today is enjoying a fair amount of popularity, and in many of the wards visited it had been introduced. However, for management within the NHS, 'The cost implications of the [this] professionalizing of nursing are certainly unwelcome' (Dingwall *et al.*, 1988, p.219). It does appear that this professionalizing strategy may not succeed for financial, rather than strategic, reasons. Also, the nursing process can be used against nurses insofar as their activities, through the reliance on documentation, become much more easily identifiable and quantifiable (Dingwall *et al.*, 1988, p.220). In this way, the 'skill-mix' of trained and untrained nurses can be altered to suit the pocket of those who hold the purse-strings.

## COUNTER-ATTACK ON INTER-PERSONAL SKILLS

Changing emphases in medical education have acted to counter the claims of nurses that they alone are interested in the patient while the medical profession is interested only in the disease. Greater emphasis is being made on training in inter-personal skills in medical education. Today, most medical schools make some attempt to cover social skills and behavioural studies in their undergraduate curriculum. It is debateable how much success that attempt is having. Many of the respondents mentioned that during their training there was relatively little input or interest in the inter-personal aspects of patient care. The unchanging emphasis on high academic qualifications for entry into medical school acts to encourage the scientifically-minded, rather than the humanistically-minded student. With the exponential growth of scientific advances in medicine, it is no bad thing that such an orientation is being sought among recruits. Questions are, however, being asked about the motivations of medical students and whether the right type of candidate is being accepted for medical school. Allen (1988, p.50) reports 'The comments made by most of the respondents who said that the main reason they wanted to study medicine was because they were good at science subjects often lacked the commitment and dedication of those who said that they had always wanted to become a doctor or to help people.' Scepticism about medical students' recruitment is also voiced by Parkhouse (1991, p.194). Perhaps, the medical student of the future will be more interested in the psychosocial aspects of health care combined with a 'scientific' bent.

The greater emphasis on inter-personal training in medical education has acted as a counter-strategy to the claims of nurses to having a different worldview and distinctive contribution to make. Nurses' attempts to establish a distinctive area of competence may not meet with success. If nurses base their claim on being caring, they are effectively arguing for doctors to be not caring: not a stance likely to appeal to members of the medical profession. But if nursing cannot establish its own area of distinctive competence, then its claims to equivalence of status will be unsuccessful. To the extent that nursing can establish the value of having different worldviews within the health care team, then as an occupation, nursing will have scored an important point.

## NURSING RESEARCH

Another attempt to improve the credibility of nursing in the eyes of the medical profession has been the encouragement of nurses to undertake research. Part of the aim has been to provide nursing with a more 'scientific' basis and move away from the unsystematized nature of nursing practice. The strategy has implicitly accepted the benefits of a scientific perspective and in turn of the inadequacies of nursing knowledge. The 'hardness' of science is preferred to the inexactitudes of practical nursing.

The knowledge-in-action (Schon, 1987) which nurses have must be systematized and catalogued – perhaps an impossible task. Medical research receives large sums of money and is well supported by various agencies, both public and private. Nursing research, however, does not have such support. Any research relies on local funding and commitment within the health authority and has, therefore, been limited in scope and size. Whether nursing research conducted under such parsimonious circumstances can actually improve the quality of nursing care is open to question.

## NURSING OFFICERS/MANAGERS

Skirmishes take place on a daily basis between the occupations: between senior nurses and doctors; Nursing Officers (now called Nurse Managers) and Consultants. House Officers have little contact with Nursing Officers but Senior Registrars have more contact with, and greater awareness of, these individuals.

The Nursing Officer acts as a link between the ward staff and the Director of Nursing Services (DNS). It is the Nursing Officer, for example, who can alert the attention of the DNS to shortages in staffing levels, problems with admissions and the number of beds. Nursing Officers often bear the brunt of the medical profession's frustrations. They are an easy target, not directly involved in clinical work and having limited power to effect changes.

Particular delight is taken by some doctors in mocking Nursing Officers for their lack of clinical involvement. The medical profession sets great store by the continued clinical involvement of even the most senior doctors. Thus, Nursing Officers are often said to be 'out of touch' and 'don't know what's going on in the wards'. They 'wander around with a handbag and a clipboard' (*Consultant*); 'people never see them' (*Consultant*); 'they are completely remote from what we do' (*Senior Registrar*) and 'they go around counting pieces of paper' (*Senior Registrar*).

In attacking Nursing Officers and the 'nursing hierarchy', the medical profession can seek to limit the power of nursing and to curtail any independence of activity among nurses. The implicit thrust of the comments about Nursing Officers was that if doctors and nurses at ward level were left to themselves, they could work quite amicably together. Doctors (and it was only doctors) found the nursing hierarchy onerous in this respect, obviously felt they could 'get round' nurses and get nurses to do whatever the doctors wanted. The implicit power struggle between senior nurses and the medical profession was occasionally made explicit:

'I think that there is a power struggle that goes on at high level as to the role of the professions, and I think that seeps down through the system to create a sense of us and them. . . .I am aware that the Sister here has a close relationship with the Nursing Officer (that she is protective of) and that we don't. We are not to go and speak to the Nursing Officer about problems, it is channelled through her. And I think that she is aspiring to be a Nursing Officer herself. And I think there is, once the nurses move away from the floor, they distance-themselves from medical staff is my perception, and there is also a perception I think of medical staff that Nursing Officers are a threat to their power base. And I think the most effective units that I have worked in are the ones where there is a strong Nursing Officer, a strong Consultant, who have mutual admiration and respect, and these units work tremendously well.' *Senior Registrar*

'The only line to the Director of Nursing Services, is through the Nursing Officer, and unless there is a close relationship there, the Nursing Officer a) doesn't appreciate exactly what the problems are, and b) you don't get the information disseminated up to the Director of Nursing Services.' *Consultant*

'I think that the nurses and the medical staff would actually work infinitely more as a team, if it wasn't for the continual interventions of the nursing hierarchy. There's a sort of feeling that the nurses' allegiance is to the nursing hierarchy rather than the doctors with whom they work, which I think would be a much better allegiance to make because that is the team that gets the patients in and out of hospital.' *Consultant*

'They certainly do not co-operate with innovations in medicine and so forth and I think that they keep the nurses down at heel a bit because they police the wards. . . . A Nursing Officer looks after so many wards and makes sure that the things in these wards are done according to her direction.' *Senior Registrar*

Nursing Officers act as a support system for nurses on the ward. Doctors do not have any similar grade looking after their interests. Indeed they do not need any such 'minders', as they appear to be quite able to look after themselves. The superior power of doctors means that nurses do need defenders. And Nursing Officers do act to protect nurses from any unreasonable demands that the medical profession might make of them. Because Nursing Officers do not work in the clinical sphere, doctors have exceedingly limited powers over them. This lack of control is obviously much resented by senior doctors and there were many comments to the effect that Nursing Officers 'should be got rid of'. This is indeed happening; there have been substantial reductions in the numbers of Nursing Officers and Nurse Managers in the last few years. This reduction is likely to continue with the establishment of Clinical Directorates. Increasing emphasis is likely to be placed on the throughput of patients and budgetary concerns than with the protection of nurses. Both the clinical autonomy of doctors and the control of nurses by Nursing Officers are likely to be diminished by the powerful limitations exerted through delegated budgets. The thorn in the side of the medical profession which Nursing Officers have sometimes provided will not have to be tolerated for long.

## OVERVIEW

In seeking to gain in occupational status, nursing is facing an uphill struggle. The medical profession is in an extremely strong position. Not only does medicine operate a very closed shop, it also enjoys considerable status and power. Medicine's relationship with the state is enviable. The circumspection with which the medical profession is treated is substantially different to the treatment that nursing receives at state level. The large size of the nursing workforce and its gender as well as its class ensures that nursing as a body will not achieve the hallowed place in the establishment which the medical profession enjoys.

However, the occupational strategies of nursing and medicine are revealing because they do demonstrate a change in the relative positions of the two. Hospitals consume a disproportionately large slice of the health care budget in the UK. The emphasis in health care is now moving albeit slowly, towards prevention and community care. The increasing acceptance of the need for change is likely to be to the advantage of nurses rather than doctors. It is, for example, nurses who are taking a leading role in stoma care and incontinence management, roles eschewed by hospital doctors.

Nurses working within the community tend to enjoy greater autonomy and independence than their hospital colleagues. Any shift in interest and resources to community care is likely to benefit nurses. It is worth noting that the medical profession itself is making attempts to establish a greater role in the community. Hospital doctors have traditionally been less interested in the rehabilitation of patients (Batchelor, 1984), but they appear to be increasingly involved in hospice work. There are now 20 rehabilitation posts in neurology in the UK, whereas ten years ago there were none (Robinson, 1991). Hospital-based doctors it seems are starting to move out of hospitals and into the community – a move which may simply underline the continuing occupational imperialism of the medical profession (Larkin, 1983, p.15). A substantial challenge to hospital medicine will be presented by the growing emphasis on costs and the evaluation of treatment options in financial terms. The measurement of outcomes will mean that general practitioners are likely to enjoy an increase in power, at the expense of hospital Consultants.

The existence of other occupational groups in health care should not be forgotten. Physiotherapists, radiographers, dieticians, social workers, occupational therapists are among the occupational groups which have impinged on the activities of both nurses and doctors. In the past, nurses for example mobilized the post-operative patient, whereas now physiotherapists will undertake that role. Doctors would have prescribed detailed diets for patients which nowadays would be the province of dieticians. Other occupational groups have emerged, and are continuing to emerge, in health care. The dominating position of doctors and the wide-ranging role of nurses are being continually challenged. More changes are likely to happen at the interfaces between new and established occupational groupings. Defences and attacks will continue in the fight for occupational space.

## Strategies and counter-strategies

In most occupations there will be strategies and counter-strategies to stave off or defend occupational territory, autonomy or position. To that extent, medicine and nursing are little different from other occupations. The strategies are of interest to those at the top of the occupation rather than those who daily carry out their work. As has been seen with nursing, there may not be consensus as to which occupational strategy should be adopted. Whose interests are to be pursued: the rank and file of an occupation, or the aspirant elite? What are the long term gains of such struggles? More money, power, status, and improved class position may be some of the goals – but for whom? It often seems that particular individuals seek fame and personal promotion by finding 'a cause' to use. Perhaps too, occupational struggles become personal struggles for those at the top. Regular dealings with the top people in the other occupation may ensure that the occupational struggle becomes a matter of personal pride to win (as in the trade union struggles of the 1960s and 1970s). Too easily can those at the top of an occupation leave behind and fail to reflect the views of the majority of members of the occupation. At the same time, the interests of senior and junior members of an occupation may differ. The professionalizing strategy in nursing and the rupture in the ranks of doctors over junior hospital doctors' hours illustrate the existence of differences within an occupation.

The occupational strategies are seldom helpful to those who consume or use the services of that occupation. All the energy expended on fending off or challenging another occupation, is energy taken away from the job in hand.

## Management

Currently, within the NHS, one other group is increasingly affecting the occupational strategies of doctors and nurses – that of *management*. The extent to which management can influence the behaviour of nurses and doctors has substantially increased over the last two years. For example, recent changes in the NHS have established Clinical Directorates in which each Unit will have its own budget. The person appointed to be the budget-holder is more likely to be a doctor than a nurse. If a nurse is the budget-holder, then the doctors will be under the overall financial direction of a nurse. As a great deal of a doctor's activities can be constrained by financial considerations, the power of a budget-holding nurse could be substantial. Similarly, if a doctor is the budget-holder then his power will be substantial. The potential to affect inter-professional relations is obvious.

Following the introduction of general management in the 1980s, nursing has lost its right to have a place at the top management level of health care. That loss may be important in affecting occupational power, as the ability to resist changes in operational activities will be correspondingly reduced. Nurses have lost managerial control over nurses (Stacey, 1988a, p.131). Thus, nurses are more likely to find themselves presented with a *fait accompli*, to which they can merely respond, rather than being in a position to initiate and follow through their own proposals. No longer will nurses views on, say, the appropriate numbers of qualified and unqualified nursing staff on a ward dominate automatically. Increasingly, decisions are being taken on the basis of statistical formulae, some of which it has to be noted, have been developed by nurses. It will be views of others, outside and with no experience of nursing, which will be heard. At the same time, nurses at ward level may find there is no one to support them or their interests at the most senior management level. The organizational changes being effected in the NHS in the 1990s mean that nursing may come to be treated as just another occupation to be budgeted for in the health care equation. Any trade-off in salary or employment conditions which nurses have made because they have a vocation for nursing will not be recognized. Their 'specialness' will be ignored. Nursing is not alone: the same situation is being faced by many occupations associated with health care.

## Quality of service; value for money

The increasing emphasis on value for money and quality of service means that the autonomy of the medical profession will be undermined as the practices of doctors come under closer scrutiny. It is a scrutiny from which 'clinical autonomy' has in the past protected the medical profession (Owens and Glennerster, 1990, p.47). The comparison through the monitoring of performances of different surgeons in relation to waiting lists, length of patient stay, use of operating theatre time, etc., means that doctors' activities will be able to be controlled. Although there is no direct assault on clinical autonomy, the scrutiny of results will be a strong management tool. Comparisons between doctors cannot aid the unity of the profession. Doctors will increasingly come to be in competition with one another.

Nurses are likely to be less affected by the changing emphasis on quality, because so much of nursing work is determined by the medical profession. Lacking the autonomy and independence of the medical profession, they have less to lose. Nevertheless, nursing is also under attack, not from the impetus to improving quality but from concerns with finance. To the extent that parts of nurses' work can be identified as not requiring nurses' particular skills, those tasks may be delegated to untrained staff. At the same time, an increasing emphasis on 'throughput' of patients may well negatively affect nurses' attachment to their work in which they may be unable to offer the quality of individual care that they would wish to give. Already, the level of motivation among nurses is not high and many are leaving, some never to return (Williams *et al.*, 1991a,b; Owens and Glennerster, 1990, p.22). Occupational and professional strategies become mere irrelevancies to those who leave the stage.

The state has always been interested in the professions in order to domesticise them (Torstendahl, 1990, p.5). Many professions are now apparently becoming too powerful for the state to tolerate. Monopolies are being eroded, traditions challenged and custom-and-practice dismissed. Recent attempts to divide the medical profession are meeting with some success. The intra-professional competition *between* doctors will be strengthened by the introduction of hospital trusts. With one hospital bidding against another, the impetus will be to shorten patient stay, increase patient throughput and find cheaper people to do the routine work. The might of the medical profession is likely to be weakened. Repeated attempts have been made to weaken many of the professions in Britain in recent years. And as Collins (1990, p.22) suggests, the history of the professions is one of decline as well as growth in power. It is no longer clear that the medical profession is still on the ascendancy. There has been a growing challenge to the perspectives of the medical profession with the advent of management and the impact of the 'internal market' in the NHS. Concern is also shifting away from the treatment of illness toward the maintenance of health, and this movement has, and will cause, more questions to be asked about the remit of the medical profession.

The concerns of many occupational groups within the NHS have for too long been inward-looking. The emphasis has been on pursuing and advancing occupational strategies. Nursing has yet to realize the benefits of its professionalizing strategies. It now seems doubtful that it ever will. Medicine, on the other hand, has done itself proud and maintained its position of pre-eminence. The challenge to nursing and medicine might now be made on behalf of the patient, who is after all both the payer and the consumer. Patients should be able to look to both nursing and medicine to defend and pursue their interests. However, the rhetoric of putting patients first has quickly been subverted by the necessity to contain costs. The cumbersome bureaucracy which once was the NHS is currently being exposed to the practices of commercial and industrial management.

# 12

# Conclusion

The National Health Service has been described as a 'collection of clubs' (Schon, 1991). The focus of this book has been to explore the relationship between two of those clubs: nursing and medicine. Neither emerges as a paragon of virtue. Despite protestations of concern about patients and the care that they are given, both occupations appear to be more interested in pursuing their own interests. Objectively it seems quite reasonable for occupational groups to be looking after themselves. However, both nursing and medicine assert that their primary interest is in working for the benefit of others, putting their own interests second. And many do, as can be attested by all those doctors and nurses who do not count the extra hours they put in on patients' behalf. Although as occupational groups there are occasional flurries of interest in protecting the interests of patients, it seems that self-interest predominates. As patients, we should not see that self-interest as reasonable. The National Health Service was designed for all of us, to be paid for by all of us, to be a service on which we could all rely to be there when we needed it. The Service has been used as a vehicle to promote occupational groupings to an unacceptable extent. The occupational strategies and professional in-fighting contrast starkly with the everyday concerns of so many nurses and doctors with their patients.

It is hard to speak out against one's own occupational group. Trouble-makers are disliked within both medicine and nursing. As 'whistle-blowers' they will be scapegoated and even lose their jobs. The present 'climate of intimidation' within the NHS effectively acts to silence anyone who speaks out. It is perhaps expecting too much of individual doctors or nurses to give voice to their reservations about the present arrangements. It may be brave, but it is also foolhardy to jeopardize a career when there is little guarantee that anything will change. As if in a quicksand, the whistle-blowers are soon covered over. There is no doubt that there is a growing need for voices to be heard. It be would admirable if real and wholehearted support could be offered by the occupational bodies to those of their members who demonstrate their wholehearted commitment to the NHS and its patients by their 'whistle-blowing'. Patients often do not have anyone to speak out on their behalf. Attempts to silence those who wish to do so, are disgraceful. Openness and accountability must be the watchwords for the future health of the NHS.

The nurses and doctors of today are some of the children who used to play imaginary 'doctors and nurses' games – grown up now and sucked into professional games about which, in their innocence, they knew nothing. The stage was already set before they arrived: they are merely transient players. These doctors and nurses are, to some extent, victims of games they never wanted to play, but having joined the team they have no option. Their way of seeing as members of one occupation is a way of **not** seeing (Hall, 1978) the other's view.

Much energy has been spent trying to find ways in which nurses and doctors could potentially work more closely. Suggestions such as sharing training, lectures, meetings, seminars, have been made.*

Mere contact is not enough, indeed it may be counterproductive, reinforcing prejudices rather than challenging them. What is required are changes in perspective and attitude. Attempts to foster such changes must be made in a systematic and comprehensive manner in order to have any impact. Those individuals who try to move away from traditional roles may simply find themselves marginalized as 'renegades' and attempts made to undermine their professional identity (Thomstad et al., 1975, p.427). The changes which are required within medicine and nursing are complementary. Nurses should be encouraged to take a year out

---

* See Baldwin, 1987; Young, 1981; Kinston, 1983; Horder et al., 1984; Mackay, 1992b.

between school and entering nursing in order to foster a self-confidence and assertiveness that has traditionally been drummed out of them. Doctors should be encouraged to take out a year between school and university in order to gain in knowledge and understanding of the lives of ordinary people. What is wanted in doctors is greater humility; what is wanted in nurses is greater pride in themselves. Of course, the professional bodies who serve themselves as much as their members, might not appreciate such changes. Such changes could mean a challenge to the received wisdom and prevailing ideologies within each occupation. The strength of the occupational socialization, on which both occupations so much depend, would be weakened. Changes such as these, which could potentially benefit the patient, will no doubt be resisted.

Doctors and nurses enter health care with a variety of different motivations, one of the strongest being to care for and look after people. Those motivations, it seems, are sometimes weakened by the organisation and priorities within the NHS. As individuals, nurses and doctors are subjects of the system they serve and the occupations of which they are members. As members of occupations they bear some measure of responsibility for the positions adopted by their occupational group. However, as individuals their power to effect any substantial change is limited.

The commitment and dedication of nurses and doctors to their patients has emerged strongly from the interviews. Nothing should be allowed to detract from their contribution to our well-being. Acting within the numerous constraints inherent in an organisation of tremendous size, doctors and nurses give us good health care. We are right to be proud of the NHS and of them. But working practices and attitudes must not become entrenched and stultifying: there is no room for complacency in health care. Nevertheless, the difficulties experienced within hospitals come from so many sources and the reasons underlying these difficulties are not simple and have no simple solution. To repeat:

'The conflicts are too complex, the issues too obscure, the cross-currents too numerous, the decisions too local to make possible the appreciation of any single formula to their solution: and it is at least reassuring some times to remember that if we found such a formula we should unquestionably be wrong. *Uno itinere no potest perveniri ad tam grande secretum.* And if we leave the subject with little more than a blurred impression in our minds we can, nonetheless, maintain that that blurred impression represents more faithfully than any clear-cut picture . . . (that which) we have been trying to understand.'*

* Collingwood and Myers, 1937.

# Appendices

## Methodology

The research was carried out within the Department of Applied Social Science, at Lancaster University. The project directors were Professor Keith Soothill and Dr. Sylvia Walby. Mrs. June Greenwell acted as research officer at various points throughout the research and was involved in conducting approximately one third of the interviews. I acted as senior research fellow, conducting two thirds of the interviews.

Interest in the research stemmed from a previous project into Nurse Recruitment and Wastage which Keith Soothill and I had undertaken, and which had resulted not only in a number of articles but also, in 1989, the book *Nursing a Problem*.

From this earlier project it appeared that many difficulties were experienced in the working relationships between nurses and doctors. On investigation we found that no systematic research had been conducted into inter-professional relations in hospitals in the UK. We decided to undertake exploratory research in this area.

We were aware that working relationships were likely to differ in various parts of the UK, and therefore sought and obtained access to five locations: three in England and two in Scotland. Teaching hospitals appeared to have a different 'atmosphere' to non-teaching, district general hospitals. Two of the locations we visited were teaching hospitals: one in Scotland and one in England, and the other three locations were District General Hospitals. At some locations there was more than one hospital, but the term 'location' has been used to cover all the associated hospitals. We were also aware that experiences were likely to be affected by the specialty in which doctors and nurses were working. We chose to focus primarily on five specialties: general medicine and general surgery – the two largest general areas within hospitals; intensive therapy; care of the elderly and psychiatry. (A deliberate decision was taken to exclude specialties in which midwives work because their situation and their history is so different from that of nurses; refer to Donnison, 1977). In some locations there were few, if any, care of the elderly beds or psychiatric beds. We then focused on two other specialties: otolaryngology and paediatrics.

### Choosing specialties

In choosing specialties we were making allowance for the influence of a number of different factors:

1. differences in length of patient stay and the throughput of patients;
2. the length of nurse training required to work in each speciality;
3. areas of care which were 'high-tech' and 'low-tech';
4. the amount of medical input into patient care;
5. high-status and low-status specialties, and,
6. to obtain a good spread of medical trainees in the different specialties from pre-registration House Officers to trainees going into general practice.

We knew from the previous research that the experience of working relationships varied with grade. We decided to include all five grades of doctor in our sample from Consultant to Junior House Officer. Because it was exploratory research we decided to confine our attentions to registered nurses, excluding untrained nursing staff and enrolled nurses.

We undertook a small pilot survey of five nurses and five doctors in a hospital in the North of England in the middle of 1989. The main survey began in the autumn of 1989 and continued until August, 1990.

We were supplied with lists of doctors and nurses working in each of the locations, in the different specialties. Respondents were selected at random, as far as possible, within each specialty. (In some specialties there may have been only one Senior Registrar and he (*sic*) would have been approached to be interviewed.)

*Interview schedules*

The interview schedule was designed to take three-quarters of an hour: in some instances, emergency and other calls meant that the interview was terminated abruptly, or was shorter than intended. Some interviews lasted for well over an hour, but the majority lasted around three-quarters of an hour to an hour. The interviews were semi-structured. There was a list of topics we sought to cover with all those interviewed, but particular topics would be explored in greater depth as appropriate. All the interviews were transcribed verbatim. Data obtained from these transcripts forms the basis of the tables within the text.

In the main survey, we carried out 135 interviews with nurses, and 127 interviews with doctors. The response rate was just over 90%, with only 28 of the 290 initially selected respondents being unable or unwilling to be interviewed. (The response rate would have been considerably higher if junior and senior House Officers did not move hospitals so frequently!) Interviews were also conducted with 17 Nursing Officers/Nurse Managers, to which only brief reference is made here. Unit General Managers were also interviewed at a later stage in the research. Contact was made and discussions held with various professional bodies, both nursing and medical.

A discussion group with a small number of final year nursing students and fourth year medical students was held in a Scottish hospital, in order to explore in greater depth some of the issues which had been identified elsewhere in the course of the interviews, and coordinated by a trained facilitator. Attempts were made, unsuccessfully, to interest the students in further joint meetings.

A small number of interviews with final year degree nurses were held, but there was an insufficient number of these, due to the timing of the interviews, to include them in our analyses. Similarly, a small number of nurses who had become

doctors were interviewed. Again, the number was too small to
include here.

## APPENDIX B. THE INTERVIEW SAMPLE

| The doctors | Male | | Female | | Total | |
|---|---|---|---|---|---|---|
| | N | % | N | % | N | % |
| Junior House Officer | 16 | 12.6 | 7 | 5.5 | 23 | 18.1 |
| Senior House Officer | 23 | 18.1 | 12 | 9.4 | 35 | 27.6 |
| Registrar | 19 | 15.0 | 9 | 7.1 | 28 | 22.0 |
| Senior Registrar | 11 | 8.7 | – | – | 11 | 8.7 |
| Consultant | 28 | 22.0 | 2 | 1.6 | 30 | 23.6 |
| Totals | 97 | 76.4 | 30 | 23.6 | 127 | 100.0 |

| The nurses | Female | | Male | | Total | |
|---|---|---|---|---|---|---|
| | N | % | N | % | N | % |
| Staff Nurse | 67 | 49.6 | 13 | 9.6 | 80 | 59.3 |
| Sister/Charge Nurse | 49 | 36.3 | 6 | 4.4 | 55 | 40.7 |
| Totals | 116 | 85.9 | 19 | 14.1 | 135 | 100.0 |

| The specialties: Doctors | Male | | Female | | Total | |
|---|---|---|---|---|---|---|
| | N | % | N | % | N | % |
| Medicine | 28 | 22.0 | 8 | 6.3 | 36 | 28.3 |
| Surgery + theatre | 24 | 18.9 | 3 | 2.4 | 27 | 21.2 |
| Otolaryngology | 10 | 7.9 | – | – | 10 | 7.9 |
| Psychiatry | 6 | 4.7 | 8 | 6.3 | 14 | 11.0 |
| Care of the elderly | 11 | 8.7 | 5 | 3.9 | 16 | 12.6 |
| Intensive Therapy Unit | 13 | 10.2 | 4 | 3.1 | 17 | 13.4 |
| Paediatrics | 5 | 3.9 | 2 | 1.6 | 7 | 5.5 |
| Totals* | 97 | 76.4 | 30 | 23.6 | 127 | 99.9 |

| The specialties: Nurses | Female | | Male | | Total | |
|---|---|---|---|---|---|---|
| | N | % | N | % | N | % |
| Medicine | 25 | 18.5 | 3 | 2.2 | 28 | 20.7 |
| Surgery + theatre | 30 | 22.2 | 3 | 2.2 | 33 | 24.4 |
| Otolaryngology | 10 | 7.4 | – | – | 10 | 7.4 |
| Psychiatry | 7 | 5.2 | 9 | 6.7 | 16 | 11.8 |
| Care of the elderly | 19 | 14.1 | 2 | 1.5 | 21 | 15.6 |
| Intensive Therapy Unit | 17 | 12.6 | 2 | 1.5 | 19 | 14.1 |
| Paediatrics | 8 | 5.9 | – | – | 8 | 5.9 |
| Totals* | 116 | 85.9 | 19 | 14.1 | 135 | 99.9 |

* Differences in totals are due to roundings.

## APPENDIX C. LENGTH OF TIME IN THE POST

|  | Doctors | | Nurses | |
|---|---|---|---|---|
|  | N | % | N | % |
| Up to 6 months | 40 | 33.6 | 13 | 10.0 |
| 6 months – 1 year | 21 | 17.6 | 18 | 13.8 |
| 1 – 2 years | 16 | 13.4 | 31 | 23.8 |
| 2 – 5 years | 19 | 16.0 | 33 | 25.4 |
| 5 – 10 years | 14 | 11.8 | 19 | 14.6 |
| > 10 years | 9 | 7.6 | 16 | 12.3 |
| Totals | 119 | 100.0 | 130 | 99.9 |

Response rate: 93.7% (doctors); 96.3% (nurses).

## APPENDIX D. FAMILIAL CONNECTIONS FOR DOCTORS AND NURSES*

|  | Doctors | | Nurses | |
|---|---|---|---|---|
|  | N | % | N | % |
| Doctor(s) | 32 | 31.7 | 6 | 5.4 |
| Nurse(s) | 13 | 12.9 | 40 | 36.0 |
| Paramedical professions | 7 | 6.9 | 2 | 1.8 |
| Unqualified health care workers | – | – | 8 | 7.2 |
| None in health care | 52 | 51.5 | 59 | 53.2 |
| Number of responses | 104 | n/a | 115 | n/a |

Response rate: 101 doctors (79.5%); 111 nurses (82.2%)
* 'Family' is used broadly to include members of the extended family: grandmothers, siblings, parents, uncles and cousins.

## APPENDIX E. 'WHAT MADE YOU DECIDE TO TAKE UP MEDICINE/NURSING?'

| | Doctors | | Nurses | |
|---|---|---|---|---|
| | N | % | N | % |
| Always wanted to | 31 | 31.0 | 52 | 41.6 |
| School performance/influence | 15 | 15.0 | 2 | 1.6 |
| Family/friends influence | 16 | 16.0 | 21 | 16.8 |
| Wanted/started another career | 15 | 15.0 | 35 | 28.0 |
| A 'good' and respected career | 13 | 13.0 | 7 | 5.6 |
| To work with people | 14 | 14.0 | 8 | 6.4 |
| Scientific element | 15 | 15.0 | 1 | 0.8 |
| Experience of illness: own/family | 4 | 4.0 | 8 | 6.4 |
| Unemployed/redundant | – | – | 4 | 3.2 |
| Other | 6 | 6.0 | 8 | 6.4 |
| | 129 | n/a | 146 | n/a |

N=100 doctors; 125 nurses
Response rate: 85.9% (225 respondents); (respondents could give more than one response).

## APPENDIX F. 'DO YOU EVER CONSIDER LEAVING MEDICINE/ NURSING?'

| | Doctors | | Nurses | |
|---|---|---|---|---|
| | N | % | N | % |
| Yes (specific job mentioned) | 21 | 25.9 | 33 | 28.7 |
| Yes, but don't know what would do | 20 | 24.7 | 30 | 26.1 |
| No | 40 | 49.4 | 52 | 45.2 |
| Totals | 81 | 100.0 | 115 | 100.0 |

Response rate: 196 respondents (74.8%).

APPENDIX G. 'WHOSE WARD DO YOU SEE IT AS BEING?'

|  | Doctors | | Nurses | |
|---|---|---|---|---|
|  | N | % | N | % |
| Sister's | 19 | 31.1 | 37 | 50.7 |
| Nurses' | 10 | 16.4 | 9 | 12.3 |
| Joint nurses'/doctors' | 8 | 13.1 | 17 | 23.3 |
| Consultant's | 14 | 22.9 | 6 | 8.2 |
| Doctor's | 2 | 3.3 | – | – |
| Nobody's | 6 | 9.8 | 3 | 4.1 |
| Patient's | 2 | 3.3 | – | – |
| Other | – | – | 1 | 1.4 |
| Totals | 61 | 99.9 | 73 | 100.0 |

Response rate: 51.1% (134 respondents); the relevance of this issue did not become apparent until the interview programme was well underway, hence low response rate.

APPENDIX H. 'WHAT NAMES DO YOU CALL EACH OTHER?'

|  | Doctors | | Nurses | |
|---|---|---|---|---|
|  | N | % | N | % |
| Surnames/titles only | 31 | 30.7 | 18 | 13.9 |
| Sister is always Sister | 24 | 23.8 | 18 | 13.9 |
| Not first names in front of patients | 14 | 13.9 | 20 | 15.5 |
| Consultants always by title | 27 | 26.7 | 78 | 60.5 |
| Senior Registrar/Registrar by title | 3 | 3.0 | 17 | 13.2 |
| Sisters call consultant by first name | 2 | 2.0 | 5 | 3.9 |
| Student nurses not called first name | 3 | 3.0 | 1 | 0.8 |
| Consultants are called by first name | 3 | 3.0 | 5 | 3.9 |
| First names | 68 | 67.3 | 105 | 81.4 |
| Consultant uses my first name | 2 | 2.0 | 16 | 12.4 |
|  | 177 | n/a | 283 | n/a |

Response rate: 87.8% (230 respondents); (respondents could give more than one response).

## APPENDIX I. 'DO YOU FEEL THAT THE DOCTORS AND NURSES WORK AS A TEAM HERE?'

|  | Doctors | | Nurses | |
|---|---|---|---|---|
|  | N | % | N | % |
| Yes | 77 | 67.5 | 77 | 58.8 |
| Sometimes/most of the time | 23 | 20.2 | 39 | 29.8 |
| No | 14 | 12.3 | 15 | 11.5 |
|  | 114 | 100.0 | 131 | 100.1 |

Response rate: 93.5% (245 respondents).

## APPENDIX J. 'DO YOU HAVE ANY SOCIAL CONTACT WITH DOCTORS/NURSES?'

|  | Doctors | | Nurses | |
|---|---|---|---|---|
|  | N | % | N | % |
| No contact | 19 | 22.1 | 25 | 22.5 |
| Occational contact | 40 | 46.5 | 50 | 45.0 |
| Yes | 27 | 31.4 | 36 | 32.4 |
| Total | 86 | 100.0 | 111 | 99.9 |

Response rate: 75.2% (197 respondents).

## APPENDIX K. 'HAVE YOU EVER BEEN ANGRY TO A NURSES'S/ DOCTOR'S FACE

|  | Yes | | No | |
|---|---|---|---|---|
|  | N | % | N | % |
| House Officers | 4 | 26.7 | 11 | 73.3 |
| Senior House Officers | 14 | 56.0 | 11 | 44.0 |
| Registrars | 14 | 66.7 | 7 | 33.3 |
| Senior Registrars | 5 | 62.5 | 3 | 37.5 |
| Consultants | 16 | 88.9 | 2 | 11.1 |
| Staff Nurses | 31 | 50.0 | 31 | 50.0 |
| Sister/Charge Nurses | 33 | 89.2 | 4 | 10.8 |

Response rate: 71.0% (87 doctors; 99 nurses).

APPENDIX L. THE EXPERIENCE OF CONFLICT IN PARTICULAR AREAS.

|  | Specific conflict | | Overt anger | | Nurses' mutter | | Doctors' mutter | | Irritation | |
|---|---|---|---|---|---|---|---|---|---|---|
|  | Doctor | Nurse | Doctor | Nurse | Doctor | Nurse | Doctor | Nurse | Doctor | Nurse |
| Calls/bleeps | 15 | 8 | 7 | 2 | 7 | 7 | 39 | 23 | 21 | 10 |
| Colleagues' attitudes | 10 | 11 | 1 | 19 | 34 | 28 | 5 | 20 | – | 27 |
| Opinions on treatment | 34 | 23 | 5 | 12 | – | – | 7 | 11 | 13 | 10 |
| Tasks not done | 13 | 12 | 12 | 4 | 6 | 12 | 12 | 15 | 11 | 15 |
| Colleagues' competence | – | – | 8 | 3 | 16 | 16 | 13 | 9 | 8 | 9 |
| Attitudes to patients | 2 | 5 | – | 12 | 17 | 16 | – | – | 1 | 21 |
| No. of respondents | 122 | 124 | 87 | 99 | 77 | 91 | 82 | 87 | 93 | 90 |
| Response rate (%) | 93.9 | | 71.0 | | 64.1 | | 64.5 | | 69.8 | |

APPENDIX M. 'DOES CALLING OUT/BEING CALLED OUT OR BLEEPING/BEING BLEEPED, CAUSE ANY PROBLEMS FOR YOU?'

|  | Doctors | | Nurses | |
|---|---|---|---|---|
|  | N | % | N | % |
| No problem | 38 | 35.9 | 56 | 50.0 |
| Yes, it can present problems | 68 | 64.1 | 56 | 50.0 |
| Number of respondents | 106 | 100.0 | 112 | 100.0 |

Response rate: 83.2% (218 respondents).

PROBLEMS INVOLVED IN BEING CALLED/CALLING AND BEING BLEEPED/BLEEPING A DOCTOR.

|  | Doctors | | Nurses | |
|---|---|---|---|---|
|  | N | % | N | % |
| Called about trivial matters | 32 | 30.2 | 19 | 17.0 |
| Doctors don't come quickly | – |  | 21 | 18.8 |
| Being woken/bleeped unpleasant | 15 | 14.2 | 5 | 4.5 |
| Doctors become angry/rude | 2 | 1.9 | 8 | 7.1 |
| Call so 'doctor informed' | 8 | 7.5 | 2 | 1.8 |
| Nurses don't have enough information when calling | 4 | 3.8 | – | – |
| Nurses can make a doctor's life miserable | 3 | 2.8 | 2 | 1.8 |
| Unspecified problem | 12 | 11.3 | 12 | 10.7 |
| More than one response per respondent | 76 | n/a | 69 | n/a |

Response rate: 83.2% (218 respondents); 106 doctors, 112 nurses.

## APPENDIX N. 'DOES TIDYING UP CAUSE ANY PROBLEMS BETWEEN DOCTORS AND NURSES?'

|  | Doctors | | Nurses | |
|---|---|---|---|---|
|  | N | % | N | % |
| Yes, it is a problem | 53 | 79.1 | 83 | 82.2 |
| No, it is not a problem | 14 | 20.9 | 18 | 17.8 |
| Number of respondents | 67 | 100.0 | 101 | 100.0 |

Response rate: 64.1% (168 respondents).

## ASPECTS OF 'TIDYING UP'

|  | Doctors | | Nurses | |
|---|---|---|---|---|
|  | N | % | N | % |
| Nurses will do it/usually do it | 14 | 20.9 | 13 | 12.9 |
| As long as you do not expect them to tidy, nurses will do it | 3 | 4.5 | 20 | 19.8 |
| Nurses ought to tidy up | 5 | 7.5 | 6 | 5.9 |
| Doctors ought to tidy up | 11 | 16.4 | 23 | 22.8 |
| I try to tidy | 28 | 41.8 | n/a | n/a |
| Some doctors do, some don't | 8 | 11.9 | 12 | 11.9 |
| If they are busy, I will tidy | 11 | 16.4 | 15 | 14.9 |
| Been told off, or left a note | 9 | 13.4 | 32 | 31.7 |
| Number of comments | 89 | n/a | 121 | n/a |

Response rate: 64.1% (168 respondents); 67 doctors, 101 nurses.

## APPENDIX O. 'WHO SHOULD BE RESPONSIBLE FOR THE ADMINISTRATION OF IV DRUGS?'

|  | Doctors | | Nurses | |
|---|---|---|---|---|
|  | N | % | N | % |
| Nurses should give IV drugs | 74 | 76.3 | 41 | 48.2 |
| Doctors should give IV drugs | 2 | 2.1 | 26 | 30.6 |
| It is not a problem for me | 8 | 8.3 | 1 | 1.2 |
| I do, or I am prepared to give IV drugs (some with reservations) | n/a | n/a | 62 | 72.9 |

Response rate: 69.5% (182 respondents); 97 doctors, 85 nurses.

## APPENDIX P. 'ARE THERE EVER ANY PROBLEMS OR DIFFERENCES OF OPINION REGARDING ISSUES SUCH AS STOPPING "ACTIVE" TREATMENT OF TERMINALLY ILL PATIENTS?'

|  | Doctors | | Nurses | |
|---|---|---|---|---|
|  | N | % | N | % |
| No problems/differences of opinion | 19 | 26.8 | 24 | 32.9 |
| Occasional problems/differences | 22 | 31.0 | 16 | 21.9 |
| Yes problems/differences of opinion | 27 | 38.0 | 26 | 35.6 |
| Nurses are asked/give their opinion | 17 | 24.0 | 28 | 38.4 |
| Nurses not asked/won't give opinion | 6 | 8.4 | 5 | 6.8 |
| It is a doctor's decision and responsibility | 25 | 35.1 | 23 | 31.6 |
| It is a joint decision | 13 | 18.3 | 18 | 24.7 |
| Doctors want to continue longer | 18 | 25.3 | 19 | 26.0 |
| Nurses want to continue longer | 5 | 7.0 | – | – |
| Total | 152 | n/a | 159 | n/a |

Response rate: 55.0% (144 respondents); 71 doctors, 73 nurses; (more than one response per respondent).

APPENDIX Q. 'IF A NURSE OFFERS AN OPINION, DO YOU FEEL
IT WILL BE LISTENED TO?'

|                    | Doctors | | Nurses | |
|                    | N | % | N | % |
|--------------------|---|---|---|---|
| Yes                | 46 | 56.8 | 40 | 36.4 |
| No                 | 2 | 2.5 | 8 | 7.3 |
| A qualified 'yes'  | 33 | 40.7 | 62 | 56.4 |
| Totals             | 81 | 100.0 | 110 | 100.1 |

Response rate: 72.9% (191 respondents).

APPENDIX R. 'DOES IT EVER HAPPEN THAT DOCTORS PRESENT
THEMSELVES AS THE "GREAT-I-AM"?'

|                        | Doctors | | Nurses | |
|                        | N | % | N | % |
|------------------------|---|---|---|---|
| Junior doctors mainly  | 35 | 48.6 | 35 | 34.0 |
| Consultants mainly     | 10 | 13.9 | 12 | 11.6 |
| A minority do          | 33 | 45.8 | 55 | 53.5 |
| The majority do        | 4 | 5.6 | 7 | 6.8 |
| Not here               | 7 | 9.7 | 14 | 14.0 |
| Totals                 | 89 | n/a | 123 | n/a |

Response rate: 66.8% (144 respondents); 72 doctors and 103 nurses: (more than
one response per respondent).

## APPENDIX S. 'ON THE WHOLE, DO YOU THINK THAT NURSES APPRECIATE THE WORK THAT DOCTORS DO?'

|  | *Doctors* | | *Nurses* | |
|---|---|---|---|---|
|  | N | % | N | % |
| Yes, on the whole I do | 22 | 20.8 | 59 | 52.7 |
| No, on the whole I do not | 23 | 21.7 | 16 | 14.3 |
| I do | – | – | 7 | 6.2 |
| I'm not sure that they do | 6 | 5.7 | 2 | 1.8 |
| Hours on call not appreciated | 34 | 32.1 | 6 | 5.4 |
| Some doctors are appreciated | 4 | 3.8 | 6 | 5.4 |
| Specific tasks mentioned only | 2 | 1.9 | 6 | 5.4 |
| Some nurses do, some don't | 15 | 14.1 | 10 | 8.9 |
|  | 106 | 100.1 | 112 | 100.1 |

Response rate: 83.2% (218 respondents).

## APPENDIX T. 'ON THE WHOLE, DO YOU THINK THAT DOCTORS APPRECIATE THE WORK THAT NURSES DO?'

|  | *Doctors* | | *Nurses* | |
|---|---|---|---|---|
|  | N | % | N | % |
| Yes, on the whole I do | 27 | 35.5 | 39 | 37.9 |
| No, on the whole I do not | 19 | 25.0 | 27 | 26.2 |
| I do | 5 | 6.6 | – | – |
| I'm not sure that they do | 1 | 1.3 | 9 | 8.7 |
| Some nurses are appreciated | 4 | 5.3 | – | – |
| Specific tasks mentioned only | 6 | 7.9 | 2 | 1.9 |
| I know from experience | 5 | 6.6 | – | – |
| Some doctors do, some don't | 9 | 11.8 | 26 | 25.2 |
| Totals | 76 | 100.0 | 103 | 99.9 |

Response rate: 68.3% (179 respondents).

## APPENDIX U. 'WHAT DO YOU THINK OF THE IDEA THAT MEDICAL STUDENTS SHOULD WORK ON THE NURSING SIDE FOR A FEW WEEKS?'

|  | Doctors | | Nurses | |
|---|---|---|---|---|
|  | N | % | N | % |
| Good idea | 34 | 34.7 | 68 | 63.0 |
| Bad idea | 10 | 10.2 | 5 | 4.6 |
| Lukewarm about the idea | 17 | 17.3 | 9 | 8.3 |
| Practical problems involved | 2 | 2.0 | – | – |
| Experiences been positive | 23 | 23.5 | 9 | 8.3 |
| Experiences been negative | 8 | 8.2 | 6 | 5.6 |
| Unsure/don't know | 4 | 4.1 | 11 | 10.2 |
| Totals | 98 | 100.0 | 108 | 100.0 |

Response rate: 78.6% (206 respondents).

## APPENDIX V. 'WHAT DO YOU THINK OF THE IDEA THAT FINAL YEAR STUDENT NURSES SHOULD SHADOW A JUNIOR DOCTOR FOR A FEW DAYS TO SEE WHAT IT WAS LIKE BEING ON CALL AND CARRYING A BLEEP?'

|  | Doctors | | Nurses | |
|---|---|---|---|---|
|  | N | % | N | % |
| Good idea | 47 | 66.2 | 43 | 62.3 |
| Bad idea | 7 | 9.9 | 14 | 20.3 |
| Lukewarm about the idea | 7 | 9.9 | 8 | 11.6 |
| Practical problems involved | 7 | 9.9 | 3 | 4.3 |
| Unsure/don't know | 3 | 4.2 | 1 | 1.4 |
| Totals | 71 | 100.1 | 69 | 99.9 |

Response rate: 53.4% (140 respondents).

## APPENDIX W. 'DO MALE NURSES HAVE A DIFFERENT RELATIONSHIP WITH DOCTORS COMPARED WITH FEMALE NURSES?'

|  | Doctors | | Nurses | |
|---|---|---|---|---|
|  | N | % | N | % |
| No difference in relationship | 56 | 46.3 | 47 | 37.6 |
| Easier relationship | 23 | 19.0 | 35 | 28.0 |
| Less easy relationship | 10 | 8.7 | 4 | 3.2 |
| Some doctors/nurses prefer female nurses | 10 | 8.7 | 13 | 10.4 |
| 'Flirty' relationship affected | 14 | 11.6 | 5 | 4.0 |
| They are more assertive/listened to | 9 | 7.4 | 21 | 16.8 |
| Homosexuality mentioned | 6 | 5.0 | 5 | 4.0 |
| Don't know any/haven't worked with | 6 | 5.0 | 14 | 11.2 |
| Totals | 134 | n/a | 144 | n/a |

Response rate: 93.9%; 121 doctors and 125 nurses; (more than one response per respondent).

## APPENDIX X. 'DO FEMALE DOCTORS HAVE A DIFFERENT RELATIONSHIP WITH NURSES COMPARED WITH MALE DOCTORS?'

|  | Doctors | | Nurses | |
|---|---|---|---|---|
|  | N | % | N | % |
| No difference in relationship | 40 | 35.4 | 74 | 56.5 |
| Easier relationship | 28 | 24.8 | 28 | 21.4 |
| Less easy relationship | 14 | 12.4 | 8 | 6.1 |
| Some doctors/nurses prefer male doctors | 27 | 23.9 | 9 | 6.9 |
| 'Flirty' relationship affected | 11 | 9.7 | 4 | 3.0 |
| They are more assertive | 4 | 3.5 | 6 | 4.6 |
| I prefer female doctors | 2 | 1.8 | 9 | 6.9 |
| They have to work harder | 16 | 14.2 | 4 | 3.0 |
| They say it is harder for them | 5 | 4.4 | – | – |
| Some specialties harder for female | 8 | 7.1 | 2 | 1.5 |
| Friction between females | 13 | 11.5 | 5 | 3.8 |
| Totals | 168 | n/a | 149 | n/a |

Response rate: 93.1%; 113 doctors and 131 nurses; (more than one response per respondent).

## COMPARISON OF FEMALE DOCTOR–NURSE RELATIONSHIPS IN SCOTLAND AND ENGLAND

| | Scotland | | | | England | | | |
| | Doctors | | Nurses | | Doctors | | Nurses | |
| | N | % | N | % | N | % | N | % |
|---|---|---|---|---|---|---|---|---|
| No difference | 14 | 29.2 | 34 | 57.6 | 26 | 40.0 | 40 | 55.6 |
| Easier relation-ship | 14 | 29.2 | 8 | 13.6 | 14 | 21.5 | 20 | 27.8 |
| Less easy relationship | 3 | 6.3 | 7 | 11.9 | 5 | 7.7 | 1 | 1.4 |
| Ease of relationship not mentioned | 17 | 35.4 | 10 | 16.9 | 20 | 30.8 | 11 | 15.3 |
| Totals | 48 | 100.1 | 59 | 100.1 | 65 | 100.1 | 72 | 100.1 |

Response rate 93.1% (244 respondents).
Differences in totals are due to roundings.

## APPENDIX Y. 'HOW DO YOU VIEW THE CHANGES IN NURSE TRAINING BROUGHT ABOUT THROUGH PROJECT 2000?'

| | Doctors | | Nurses | |
| | N | % | N | % |
|---|---|---|---|---|
| Overall, a good idea | 20 | 18.7 | 50 | 39.7 |
| Overall, a bad idea | 51 | 47.7 | 35 | 27.8 |
| Overall, uncertain | 29 | 27.1 | 38 | 30.1 |
| Don't know enough about it | 7 | 6.5 | 3 | 2.4 |
| Totals | 107 | 100.0 | 126 | 100.0 |

Response rate 88.9% (233 respondents).

'WILL THE PROJECT 2000 CHANGES MAKE ANY DIFFERENCE TO INTER-PROFESSIONAL RELATIONSHIPS BETWEEN NURSES AND DOCTORS?'

| | Doctors | | Nurses | |
|---|---|---|---|---|
| | N | % | N | % |
| Nurses will be less practical/ less practically experienced | 43 | 40.2 | 34 | 27.0 |
| Doctors will see nurses as professionals | 4 | 3.7 | 28 | 22.2 |
| Won't change doctors' view of nurses | 16 | 14.9 | 13 | 10.3 |
| Nurses will be more assertive | 4 | 3.6 | 16 | 12.7 |
| Nurses will be more knowledgeable | 16 | 14.9 | 14 | 11.1 |
| Nurses will challenge doctors more | 14 | 13.1 | 10 | 7.9 |
| Nurses will be unwilling to do basic nursing | 10 | 9.3 | 1 | 0.8 |
| Will lose students/numbers on ward | 8 | 7.5 | 14 | 11.1 |
| Graduate nurses are seen negatively | 2 | 1.9 | 4 | 3.2 |
| Totals | 117 | n/a | 134 | n/a |

Response rate 88.9%: 107 doctors, 126 nurses; (more than one response per respondent).

## APPENDIX Z. COMMENTS ON THE ROLE OF THE NURSE

| | Doctors | | Nurses | |
|---|---|---|---|---|
| | N | % | N | % |
| It should be greater | 56 | 75.7 | 36 | 61.0 |
| It should stay as it is | 10 | 13.5 | 11 | 18.6 |
| Uncertain | 8 | 10.8 | 12 | 20.3 |
| Totals | 74 | 100.0 | 59 | 99.9 |

Response rate: 50.8%

# References

Abel-Smith, B. (1960) *A History of the Nursing Profession*, Heinemann, London.

Allan, D. (1989) Brain death. *Nursing Times*, **85** (35), 30–2.

Allen, I. (1988) *Doctors and their Careers*, Policy Studies Institute, London.

Armstrong, D. (1983) The Fabrication of Nurse-Patient Relationships. *Social Science and Medicine*, **17** (8), 457–60.

Ashley, J.A. (1980) Power in Structured Misogeny. *Advances in Nursing Science*, **2** (3), 3.

Atkinson, P.A. (1976) Upstairs, downstairs: medical students in their first clinical year and their previous experience in hospitals. *Medical Education*, **10**, 3–9.

Atkinson, P. (1977) The Reproduction of Medical Knowledge. In *Health Care and Health Knowledge*, (ed. R. Dingwall), Croom Helm, London, pp.85–106.

Baldwin, A., Welches, L., Walker, D.D. and Eliamstam, M. (1987) Nurse self-esteem and collaboration with physicians. *Western Journal of Nursing Research*, **9**, 107–14.

Baly, M.E. (1986) *Florence Nightingale and the Nursing Legacy*, Croom Helm, London.

Batchelor, I. (1984) In *Hospital Medicine and Nursing in the 1980s: Interaction between the professions of medicine and nursing*, (eds. A. Duncan and G. McLachlan), Nuffield Provincial Hospitals Trust, London.

Bates, B. (1966a) Nurse Physician Teamwork, Part 1. *International Nursing Review*, **13** (5), 43–54.

Bates, B. (1966b) Nurse Physician Teamwork, Part 2. *International Nursing Review*, **13** (6), 53–61.

Becker, H.S., Geer, B., Hughes, E.C. and Strauss, A.S. (1961) *Boys in White*, Transaction Books, New Brunswick, Reprinted 1983.

Beechey, V. and Perkins, T. (1987) *A Matter of Hours*, Polity Press, Cambridge.

Bell, E.M. (1953) *Storming the Citadel, the Rise of the Woman Doctor*, Constable, London.

Bellaby, P. and Oribabor, P. (1980) The History of the Present

Contradiction and Struggle in Nursing. In *Rewriting Nursing History*, (ed. C. Davies), Croom Helm, London, pp.147–74.

Benner, P. (1984) *From Novice to Expert*, Addison-Wesley, Menlo Park, California.

Berlant, J.L. (1975) *Profession and Monopoly: A Study of Medicine in the United States and Great Britain*, University of California Press, Berkeley, Los Angeles.

Birch, J. (1975) *To Nurse or Not to Nurse: An Investigation into the Causes of Withdrawal During Nurse Training*, Royal College of Nursing, London.

Blanche, G. (1988) Doctors, Despite it all: Stresses in Medical Training. *Holistic Medicine*, **3**, 151–60.

Bond, J. and Bond, S. (1980) *Sociology and Health Care*, Churchill Livingstone, London.

Bowers, D.M. (1970) Why Not Teach Nursing to Doctors? *Nursing Times*, **66** (24), 24.

Bowling, A. (1981) *Delegation in General Practice: A Study of Doctors and Nurses*, Tavistock, London.

Bradley, H. (1989) *Men's Work, Women's Work*, Polity Press, Cambridge.

Bradshaw, J.S. (1978) *Doctors on Trial*, Paddington Press, New York.

Bradshaw, P.L. (1984) A Quaint Philosophy. *Senior Nurse*, **1** (35), 11.

Brazell, H. (1987) Doctors as Managers. *Management Education and Development*, **18** (2), 95–102.

British Medical Association (1981) *The Handbook of Medical Ethics*, British Medical Association, London.

Brown, R.G.S. and Stones, R.W.H. (1973) *The Male Nurse*, G. Bell, London.

Burns, T. (1953) Friends, Enemies and Polite Fiction. *American Sociological Review*, **18**, December, 654–62.

Campbell-Heider, N. and Pollock, D. (1987) Barriers to Physician-Nurse Collegiality: An Anthropological Perspective. *Social Science and Medicine*, **25** (5), 421–5.

Carpenter, M. (1978) Managerialism and the division of labour in nursing. In *Readings in the Sociology of Nursing*, (eds. R. Dingwall and J. McIntosh), Churchill Livingstone, Edinburgh.

Carpenter, M. (1977) The New Managerialism and Professionalism in Nursing. In *Health and the Division of Labour*, (eds. M. Stacey and M. Reid), Croom Helm, London.

Castledine, G. (1981) The nurse as the patient's advocate – pros and cons. *Nursing Mirror*, **153** (20), 38–40.

Central Statistical Office (1991) *Regional Trends*, **26**, HMSO, London.

Central Statistical Office (1992) *Annual Abstract of Statistics*, No.128, HMSO, London.

Chapman, C.M. (1977) Image of the nurse. *International Nursing Review*, **24**, 166–70.

Clark, M.O. (1984) In *Hospital Medicine and Nursing in the 1980s:*

*Interaction between the professions of medicine and nursing*, (eds. A. Duncan and G. McLachlan), Nuffield Provincial Hospitals Trust, London.

Cockburn, C. (1988) The Gendering of jobs: workplace relations and the reproduction of sex segregation. In *Gender Segregation at Work*, (ed. S. Walby), Open University Press, Milton Keynes, pp.29–42.

Collingwood, R.G. and Myers, J.N.L.(1937) (Second edition) *Roman Britain and the English Settlements*, Oxford University Press, Oxford.

Collins, R. (1990) Changing conceptions in the sociology of the professions. In *The Formation of Professions: Knowledge, State and Society*, (eds. R. Torstendahl and M. Burrage), Sage, London, pp.11–23.

Community Relations Commission (1976) *Doctors from Overseas, a Case for Consultation*, Community Relations Commission, London.

Conway, M.E. (1983) Socialization and Roles in Nursing. *Annual Review of Nursing Research*, 1, 183–208.

Coser, R.L. (1972) Authority and Decision-Making in a Hospital: A Comparative Analysis. In *Medical Men and Their Work*, (eds. E. Freidson and J. Lorber), Aldine Atherton, Chicago pp.174–84.

Crowley, S.A. and Wollner, I.S. (1987) Collaborative Practice: A Tool for Change. *Oncology Nursing Forum*, 14 (4), 59–63.

Darbyshire, P. (1987) The burden of history. *Nursing Times*, 83 (4), 32–4.

Davidson, N. (1987) *A Question of Care: the changing face of the National Health Service*, Michael Joseph, London.

De la Cuesta (1983) The nursing process: from development to implementation. *Journal of Advanced Nursing*, 8 (5), 365–71.

Delamothe, T. (1988a) Nursing Grievances: Pay and agency nurses. *British Medical Journal*, 296, 120–3.

Delamothe, T. (1988b) Nursing Grievances: Not a profession, not a career. *British Medical Journal*, 296, 271–4.

Department of Health (1990) *Consultants' Distinction Awards*, Department of Health, London.

Department of Health (1992) Personal communication.

Dingwall, R., Rafferty, A.M. and Webster, C. (1988) *An Introduction to the Social History of Nursing*, Routledge, London.

Doggett, M-A. (1988) Women Doctors and their Careers: A Review of the Literature. In *Doctors and their Careers*, I. Allen, Policy Studies Institute, London, Appendix B.

Donnison, J. (1977) *Midwives and Medical Men: A History of Interprofessional Rivalries and Women's Rights*, Heinemann, London.

Dowie, R. (1987) *Postgraduate medical education and training: the system in England and Wales*, Oxford University Press, King Edward's Hospital Fund, London.

Duncan, A.S. (1984) In *Hospital Medicine and Nursing in the 1980s: Interaction between the professions of medicine and nursing*, (eds. A. Duncan and G. McLachlan), Nuffield Provincial Hospitals Trust, London.

Dyer, C. (1991) Raw deal for sisters in law. *The Guardian*, 15th May, p.21.

Ehrenreich, B. and English, D. (1973) *Witches, Midwives and Nurses: A history of women healers*, Feminist Press, New York.

Elston, M.A. (1977a) Women in the Medical Profession: Whose problem? In *Health and the Division of Labour*, (eds. M. Stacey and M. Reid), Croom Helm, London, pp.116–34.

Elston, M.A. (1977b) Medical Autonomy: the Challenge and Response. In *Conflict in the National Health Service*, (eds. K.A.B. Barnard and K. Lee), Croom Helm, London, Chapter 2.

Etzioni, A. (ed) (1969) *The Semi-Professions and Their Organization*, Free Press, New York.

Festinger, L. (1957) *A Theory of Cognitive Dissonance*, Row Peterson, Evanston, Illinois.

Field, D. (1984) Formal Instruction in United Kingdom medical schools about death and dying. *Medical Education*, **18**, 429–34.

Field, D. (1989) *Nursing the Dying*, Routledge, London.

Firth, J. (1986) Levels and sources of stress in medical students. *British Medical Journal*, **292**, 1177–80.

Firth-Cozens, J. (1987) Emotional distress in junior house officers. *British Medical Journal*, **295**, 533–6.

Foucault, M. (1973) *The Birth of the Clinic*, Tavistock, London.

Francis, B., Peelo, M. and Soothill, K. (1992) NHS nursing: career, vocation or just a job? In *Themes and Perspectives in Nursing*, (eds. K. Soothill, C. Hendry and K. Kendrick), Chapman & Hall, London.

Freidson, E. (1970a) *Profession of Medicine*, Dodd, Mead, New York.

Freidson, E. (1970b) *Professional Dominance*, Atherton, New York.

Furnham, A.F. (1986) Medical students' beliefs about nine different specialties. *British Medical Journal*, **293**, 1607–10.

Furnham, A., Pendleton, D. and Manicom, C. (1981) The perception of different occupations within the medical profession. *Social Science and Medicine*, **15E**, 289–300.

Gamarnikow, E. (1978) Sexual Division of Labour: The Case of Nursing. In *Feminism and Materialism*, (eds. A. Kuhn and A. Wolpe), Routledge and Kegan Paul, London, pp.96–123.

Gardner, H. and McCoppin, B. (1986) Vocation, career or both? *Australian Journal of Advanced Nursing*, **4** (1), 25–35.

Gaze, H. (1987) Man Appeal. *Nursing Times*, **83** (30), 24–7.

Glaser, B.G. and Strauss, A.L. (1968) *The Discovery of Grounded Theory*, Weidenfeld and Nicholson, London.

Goffman, E. (1969) *The Presentation of Self in Everyday Life*, Penguin, Harmondsworth.

Gouldner, A.W. (1957) Cosmopolitans and Locals. *Administrative Science Quarterly*, **2**, 281–306.

Green, S. (1974) *The Hospital: An Organizational Analysis*, Blackie, Glasgow.

Hakim, C. (1991) Grateful slaves and self-made women: fact and fantasy in women's work orientations. *European Sociological Review*, **7** (2), 101–21.

Hall, D.U. (1978) 'What nurse don't see, she don't worry about', or the use of observation in hospital research. *Nursing Times, Occasional Paper*, **74** (34), 137–40.

Hardy, L. (1987) The Male Model. *Nursing Times*, **83** (21), 36–8.

Harris, C.M. (1981) Medical Stereotypes. *British Medical Journal*, **283**, 1676–7.

Hart, L. (1991) A Ward of my Own: Social Organisation and Identity among Hospital Domestics. In *Anthropology and Nursing*, (eds. P. Holden and J. Littlewood), Routledge, London.

Heenan, A. (1991) Uneasy Partnership. *Nursing Times*, **87** (10), 25–7.

Heiberg, A.N. (1987) The doctor in the twenty-first century. *British Medical Journal*, **295**, 1602–3.

Horder, J., Ellis, J. and Hirsch, S., *et al.* (1984) An important opportunity: An open letter to the General Medical Council. *British Medical Journal*, **288**, 1507–11.

Horsley, J.E. (1987) A hostile doctor? *RN*, April, 77–8.

Hughes, D. (1988a) Subtle Decision-Making. *Nursing Times*, **84** (22), 52.

Hughes, D. (1988b) When nurse knows best: some aspects of nurse/doctor interaction in a casualty department. *Sociology of Health and Illness*, **10** (1), 1–22.

Illich, I. (1977) *Limits to Medicine, Medical Nemesis: the Expropriation of Health*, Penguin, Harmondsworth.

Illman, J. (1989) Short-cut to the bypass surgeon's scalpel. *The Guardian*, 15th September, p.24.

James, N. (1989) Emotional labour: skills and work in the social regulation of feelings. *Sociological Review*, **37** (1), 15–42.

Johnson, T.J. (1972) *Professions and Power*, Macmillan, London.

Johnson, M.L. (1971a) A comparison of the social characteristics and academic achievement of medical students and unsuccessful medical school applicants. *British Journal of Medical Education*, **5** (4), 260–3.

Johnson, M.L. (1971b) Non-academic factors in medical school selection. *British Journal of Medical Education*, **5** (4), 264–8.

Johnson, M. (1978) Big fleas have little fleas – nurse professionalisation and nursing auxiliaries. In *Nursing Auxiliaries in Health Care*, (eds. M. Hardie and L. Hockey), Croom Helm, London, pp.103–17.

Jolley, M. (1989) The Professionalization of Nursing: the Uncertain Path. In *Current Issues in Nursing*, (eds. M. Jolley and P. Allan), Chapman & Hall, London, pp.1–22.

Kalisch, B.J. and Kalisch, P. (1977) An Analysis of the sources of physician-nurse conflict. *Journal of Nursing Administration*, **7** (1), 51–7.

Kalisch, P.A. and Kalisch, B.J. (1986) A comparative analysis of nurse and physician characters in the entertainment media. *Journal of Advanced Nursing*, **11**, 179–95.

Katz, F.E. (1969) Nurses. In *The Semi-Professions and their Organization*, (ed. A. Etzioni), Free Press, New York.

Kerr, J.A.C. (1986) Interpersonal distance of hospital staff. *Western Journal of Nursing Research*, **8** (3), 350–64.

Kerrison, S. (1990) *A diplomat in the job: Diabetes Nursing and the changing division of labour in diabetic care*, South Bank Polytechnic, Health and Social Services Research Unit, Research Paper 4, London.

Kinston, W. (1983) Hospital organisation and structure and its effects on inter-professional behaviour and the delivery of care. *Social Science and Medicine*, **17** (16), 1159–70.

Larson, M.S. (1977) *The Rise of Professionalism, a Sociological Analysis*, University of California Press, Berkeley and Los Angeles.

Larkin, G. (1983) *Occupational Monopoly and Modern Medicine*, Tavistock, London.

Lawler, J. (1991) *Behind the Screens: Nursing, Somology and The Problem of the Body*, Churchill Livingstone, Edinburgh.

Lawrence, B. (1987) The Fifth Dimension – Gender and General Practice. In *In a Man's World*, (eds. A. Spencer and D. Podmore), Tavistock, London, pp.134–57.

Leeson, J. and Gray, J. (1978) *Women and Medicine*, Tavistock, London.

Lepenies, W. (1988) *Between Literature and Science: the Rise of Sociology*, Cambridge University Press, Cambridge.

Lester, E. (1986) Personal View. *British Medical Journal*, **293**, 331.

Loftus, G.T. (1971) Differential Conceptions of Physician Responsibility. *Journal of Medical Education*, **46** (4), 290–8.

Lorber, J. (1984) *Women Physicians: Careers, status and power*, Tavistock, London/New York.

Lovell, M.C. (1981) Silent but perfect 'partners': Medicine's use and abuse of women. *Advances in Nursing Science*, **3** (1), 25–40.

Mackay, L. (1989) *Nursing a Problem*, Open University Press, Milton Keynes.

Mackay, L. and Torrington, D. (1986) *The Changing Nature of Personnel Management*, Institute of Personnel Management, London.

Mackay, L. (1992a) Nursing and doctoring: where's the difference? In *Themes and Perspectives in Nursing*, (eds. K. Soothill, C. Henry and K. Kendrick), Chapman & Hall, London.

Mackay, L. (1992b) Working and cooperating in hospital practice. *Journal of Interprofessional Care*, **6** (2), 127–31.

Mackie, R.E. (1967) Family problems in medical and nursing families. *British Journal of Medical Psychology*, **40** (4), 333–40.

McAuley, J. (1987) Women Academics: A Case Study in Inequality. In *In a Man's World*, (eds. A. Spencer and D. Podmore), Chapter 8.

McCormick, J. (1979) *The Doctor: Father Figure or Plumber?*, Croom Helm, London.

McKeown, T. (1976) *The Role of Medicine: dream, mirage or nemesis?* Nuffield Provincial Hospitals Trust, London.

McPherson, A. and Small, J. (1980) Women GPs in Oxfordshire. *Journal of the Royal College of General Practitioners*, **30**, 108–11.

Maclean, U. (1974) *Nursing in Contemporary Society*, Routledge and Kegan Paul, London.

Marinker, M. (1974) Medical Education and Human Values. *Journal of the Royal College of General Practitioners*, **24**, 445–62.

Martin, J.P. (1984) *Hospitals in Trouble*, Blackwell, Oxford.

Melia, K. (1984) Student nurses' construction of occupational socialisation. *Sociology of Health and Illness*, **6** (2), 132–51.

Melia, K. (1987) *Learning and Working: The Occupational Socialization of Nurses*, Tavistock, London.

Menzies, I. (1970) *The Functioning of Social systems as a Defence Against Anxiety*, Tavistock, Centre for Applied Social Research.

Millman, M. (1976) *The Unkindest Cut: Life in the Backrooms of Medicine*, M. Morrow, New York.

Mills, W. (1983) *Problems related to the nursing management of the dying patient*, University of Glasgow, M. Litt. Thesis.

Mitchell, T. (1984) Is nursing any business of doctors? *Nursing Times*, **80** (19), 28–32.

Newby, H. (1975) The deferential dialectic. *Comparative Studies in History and Society*, **17** (2), April, 139–64.

Owens, P. and Glennerster, H. (1990) *Nursing in Conflict*, Macmillan, Basingstoke.

Parkhouse, J. (1991) *Doctors; Careers, Aims and Experiences of Medical Graduates*, Routledge, London.

Parry, N. and Parry, J. (1976) *The Rise of the Medical Profession*, Croom Helm, London.

Phillips, M. (1991) Damning of a doctor. *The Guardian*, 10th May, p.19.

Pigache, P. (1991) Being a doctor can injure your health. *The Guardian*, 4th October, p.29.

Pringle, R. (1988) *Secretaries Talk*, Veso, London/New York.

Reeve, P.E. (1980) Personality characteristics of a sample of anaesthetists. *Anaesthesia*, **35**, 559–68.

Reilly, B.J. and Di Angelo, J.A. (1990) Communication: a cultural system of meaning and value. *Human Relations*, **43** (2), 129–40.

Revans, R.W. (1962) Hospital Attitudes and Communications. In *Sociological Review Monograph No.5 Sociology and Medicine*, (ed. P. Halmos), University of Keele, Keele, pp.117–43.

Rezler, A.G. (1974) Attitude changes during Medical School: A Review of the Literature. *Journal of Medical Education*, **49**, 1023–30.

Richards, P. (1983) *Learning Medicine*, British Medical Association, London.

Roberts, S. (1983) Oppressed group behavior: implications for nursing. *Advanced Nursing Science*, **6**, 21–30.

Robinson, I. (1991) *Reframing rehabilitation: the reorientation of medical knowledge*. Paper presented at the British Sociological Association Conference, Manchester, 25th–28th March.

Robinson, J. (1986a) Covering up for the doctor. *Nursing Times*, **82** (30), 35–6.

Robinson, J. (1986b) Through the minefield – and into the sun? *Senior Nurse*, **4** (6), 7–9.

Robinson, J. (1989) Nursing in the Future: A Cause for Concern. In

*Current Issues in Nursing,* (eds. M. Jolley and P. Allan), Chapman & Hall, London.

Runciman, P.J. (1983) *Ward Sister at Work,* Churchill Livingstone, Edinburgh.

Sacks, O. (1986) *A Leg to Stand On,* Pan, London.

Salvage, J. (1985) *The Politics of Nursing,* Heinemann, London.

Scase, R. and Goffee, R. (1989) *Reluctant Managers: Their Work and Lifestyles,* Unwin Hyman, London.

Schmitt, M.H. and Williams, T.F. (1985) Nurse-physician Collaboration and Outcomes for Patients. *Annals of Internal Medicine,* **103** (6), 956.

Schon, D. (1987) *Educating the Reflective Practitioner,* Jossey Bass, San Francisco.

Schon, D. (1991) Reflective Practice and Phenomenology; conference address, *Interprofessional Collaboration: The Vision and the Challenge,* King's Fund Centre, London, 20th June.

Skeet, M. and Elliott, K. (eds.) (1978) *Health Auxiliaries and the Health Team,* Croom Helm, London.

Smith, D.J. (1980) *Overseas doctors in the National Health Service,* Heinemann Educational Books/Policy Studies Institute, London.

Smith, L. (1987a) Doctors Rule, OK? *Nursing Times,* **83** (30), 49–51.

Smith, T. (1987b) Clinical freedom. *British Medical Journal,* **295**, 1583.

Soothill, K. and Bradby, M. (1992) *Ever Considered Being a Doctor?* Unpublished working paper, University of Lancaster.

Spencer, A. and Podmore, D. (1987) Women Lawyers – Marginal Members of a Male-Dominated Profession. In *In a Man's World,* (eds. A. Spencer and D. Podmore), Tavistock, London.

Stacey, M. (1985) Women and Health: the United States and the United Kingdom compared. In *Women, Health and Healing,* (eds. E. Lewin and V. Olesen), Tavistock, New York, pp.270–97.

Stacey, M. (1988a) *The Sociology of Health and Healing,* Unwin Hyman, London.

Stacey, M. (1988b) Power, responsibility and accountability: a critical analysis of the British Medical profession. *Medical Sociology News,* **14** (1), 10–39.

Stein, L. (1967) The doctor–nurse game. *Archives of General Psychiatry,* **16**, 699–703.

Stein, L., Watts, D. and Howell, T. (1990) The doctor–nurse game revisited. *New England Journal of Medicine,* **322** (8), 546–9.

Strong, P. and Robinson, J. (1988) *New Model Management: Griffiths and the NHS,* University of Warwick, Nursing Policy Studies, No. 3.

Strong, P. and Robinson, J. (1990) *The NHS: Under New Management,* Open University Press, Buckingham.

Tellis-Nyak, M. and Tellis-Nyak, V. (1984) Games that Professionals Play: the social psychology of physician-nurse interaction. *Social Science and Medicine,* **18** (12), 1063–9.

Thomstad, B., Cunningham, N. and Kaplan, B.H. (1975) Changing the Rules of the Doctor–Nurse Game. *Nursing Outlook,* **23** (7), 422–7.

Torstendahl, R. (1990) Introduction: promotion and strategies of knowledge based groups. In *The Formation of Professions: Knowledge, State and Strategy*, (eds. R. Torstendahl and M. Burrage), Sage, London, pp.1–10.

Tuckett, D.(ed) (1976) *An Introduction to Medical Sociology*, Tavistock, London.

Turner, B.S. (1987) *Medical Power and Social Knowledge*, Sage, London.

United Kingdom Central Council (1987) *Project 2000: The Final Proposals*, UKCC, Project Paper 9, London.

United Kingdom Central Council (1991) The scope of professional practice. *Register*, Spring, p.7.

Uprichard, M. (1971) Ferment in Nursing. *International Nursing Review*, **16** (3), 222–4.

Vachon, M.L.S. (1978) Motivation and Stress Experienced by Staff Working with the Terminally Ill. *Health Education*, **2**, 113–22.

Waite, R. and Hutt, R. (1987) *Attitudes, Jobs and Mobility of Qualified Nurses: A Report for the Royal College of Nursing*, University of Sussex, Institute of Manpower Studies, IMS Report No. 130.

Wakeford, R.E. and Allery, L. (1986) Doctors' attitudes, medical philosophy, and political views. *British Medical Journal*, **292**, 1025–7.

Watkins, S. (1987) *Medicine and Labour: the politics of a profession*, Lawrence and Wishart, London.

Webster, D. (1985) Medical students' views of the nurse. *Nursing Research*, **34** (5), 313–7.

Whitehouse, C.R. (1986) Conflict and cooperation between doctors and nurses in primary health care. *Nursing Practice*, **1** (4), 242–5.

Williams, C. (1991a) Love nursing, hate the job. *The Health Service Journal*, **101** (5238), 18–21.

Williams, C. (1991b) Targeting the discontented. *The Health Service Journal*, **101** (5239), 20–1.

Willis, E. (1983) *Medical Dominance: The division of labour in Australian health care*, Allen and Unwin, Sydney.

Wilson, R.N. (1954) Teamwork in the Operating Room. *Human Organization*, **12**, 9–14.

Wolf, Z.R. (1986) Nurses' work: the sacred and the profane. *Holistic Nursing Practice*, **1** (1), 29–35.

Woolley, H., Stein, A., Forrest, G.C., and Baumn, J.D. (1989) Staff stress and job satisfaction at a children's hospice. *Archives of Disease in Childhood*, **64**, 114–8.

Young, G. (1981) A Woman in Medicine: Reflections from the Inside. In *Women, Health and Reproduction*, (ed. H. Roberts), Routledge and Kegan Paul, London, pp.144–62.

# Author index

# Subject index

Absenteeism 18–19, 83, 85
Academic
  and medical profession 37, 42,
    43, 138, 165, 166, 247
  and nursing 42, 164, 211, 217
Active treatment, of terminally ill
    45, 60, 140, 143, 146, 149–52
  *see also* Dying patients
Admission of patients 29, 64, 66,
    71, 90, 138, 249
Agency nurses 83–5, 119, 199
Allegiance, of consultant and
    sister 65–6
  *see also* Loyalty
Alliances 226
  *see also* Loyalty
Anger, displayed 144–7, 122–3,
    131, 145, 176–7, 188, 224
Anti-intellectual 42
Anti-professional 244
Anti-women views 200
Appreciation,
  of work of others 58–9, 82,
    97–8, 119, 123, 125, 127, 170,
    185–6, 219, 220, 221, 245
  lack of 123, 186, 188–9
Areas of competence, nurses
    attempt to establish 71, 236,
    248
Assertiveness, nurses 211
Assistant doctor, nurse as 4
Atmosphere
  in nursing 41, 219
  ward 29–31, 80–2, 84, 87–8,
    107, 109
Attitudes
  to colleagues 2, 50, 94, 106,

115, 117, 119–20, 177–8,
  187–90, 194
to patients 84, 117, 166, 167–8
*see also* View of doctor; View of
  nurses
Auxiliaries, nurses 38–9, 109, 121,
  144, 155, 236, 237, 243
plans to phase out 218

Backgrounds
  of doctors 16
  of nurses 16
  *see also* Class
Bank nurses 83
Blood pressure, taking 124–33,
  138
Blood samples ('taking blood') 31,
  129, 133, 240–1
'Born not made', nurses 52, 165
  *see also* Vocation
British Medical Association
  (BMA) 234, 241
  *see also* Professional Bodies

Care of the terminally ill 45, 116,
  139–60, 168, 230, 237
  *see also* Dying Patients
Career choice, *see* Occupational
  choice
Career
  medical 35–6, 45–7, 52–3, 96,
    153–5, 172, 202, 228, 230,
    232
    successful 23, 34
    and women doctors 54–5,
      197–204

## Conflicts in Care
## Medicine and Nursing
Lesley Mackay

Based on unique research at a variety of hospitals in England and Scotland, this text considers the everyday working relationships between doctors and nurses.

It explores the dynamics of this relationship and the effect not only on the nurses and doctors but on their patients. The book is based on the views of doctors and registered nurses of all grades: exploring and taking delight in the complexities of these relationships.

It can be used as a checklist for good practice or maximizing co-operation but it also warns against simplistic solutions. The writing is clear and jargon free.

*Conflicts in Care* will be of interest to practising doctors and nurses, students, and health care managers. In particular, the book will be of interest to all concerned with the quality of health care currently being provided in hospitals.

Dr Lesley Mackay has been a professional researcher for over ten years, and is currently Senior Research Fellow in the Department of Applied Social Science, Lancaster University, UK.

### Also available

**Stress and Coping in Nursing**
R. Bailey and M. Clark
Paperback (0 412 33830 0), 352 pages

**Challenges in Caring**
**Explorations in nursing and ethics**
James M. Brown, Alison L. Kitson and Terence J. McK
Paperback (0 412 34400 9), 236 pages

**Current Issues in Nursing**
Moya Jolley and Peta Allan
Paperback (0 412 32850 X), 184 pages

**Themes and Perspectives in Nursing**
Edited by Keith Soothill, Christine Henry and Kevin Kendrik
Paperback (0 412 43990 5), 348 pages

E6 1993
NOTTINGHAM UNIVERSITY BOOKSHOP
£13.95

## CHAPMAN & HALL
London · Glasgow · New York · Tokyo · Melbourne · Madras

Co-published in the United States with Singular Publishing Group Inc., San Diego, California.
ISBN 1–56593–120–3 (USA only)

ISBN 0-412-47860-9

9 780412 4786